D1454608

Health and
Wealth

Health and Wealth

An International Study of Health-Care Spending

Robert J. Maxwell

Published for
Sandoz Institute for
Health and Socio-Economic
Studies

by

LexingtonBooks
D.C. Heath and Company
Lexington, Massachusetts
Toronto

This international comparative study was done by Robert J. Maxwell for and in collaboration with the Sandoz Institute for Health and Socio-Economic Studies in Geneva. The designations employed and the presentation of material in this publication do not imply the expression of any opinion whatsoever on the part of the Sandoz Institute concerning the legal status of any country, territory, city, or area or of its authorities, or concerning the delimitation of its frontiers or boundaries. The designations used are essentially those indicated in the literature from which the data were retrieved.

Library of Congress Cataloging in Publication Data

Maxwell, Robert J
    Health and wealth.

    Bibliography: p.
    Includes index.
    1. Medical care, Cost of. 2. Medical care, Cost of—Statistics. I. Title.
[DNLM: 1. Costs and cost analysis. 2. Expenditures, Health. W74 M465h]
RA410.M38   338.4'33621   80-8427
ISBN 0-669-04109-2

Copyright © 1981 by D.C. Heath and Company

All rights reserved. No part of this publication may be reproduced or transmitted in any form or by any means, electronic or mechanical, including photocopy, recording, or any information storage or retrieval system, without permission in writing from the publisher.

Fourth printing, November 1983

Published simultaneously in Canada

Printed in the United States of America

International Standard Book Number: 0-669-04109-2

Library of Congress Catalog Card Number: 80-8427

Contents

                Included in the Survey   121

Appendix D   **Bibliographical References**   169

                Index   175

                About the Author   180

List of Figures

List of Tables

Foreword

Twenty years ago, spending on health care was a subject that attracted little international interest. During 1979, it was the subject of no fewer than six international conferences and seminars, with further international discussions scheduled for 1980.

The recent concentration of interest in the subject is simply explained. Estimates for the mid-1950s suggested that highly industrialized countries tended to spend around 4 percent of their resources on health care. The estimates for ten such countries for 1977 are presented by Robert Maxwell in this volume. They show three countries (Sweden, West Germany, and the United States) spending between 9 and 10 percent, and six others spending between 6.4 and 8.2 percent of gross national product (GNP) on health care. Only one country (the United Kingdom) was substantially below these figures, at 5.2 percent. When national economies were growing rapidly, the fact that spending on health care was growing faster than GNP did not cause great concern. But with the much lower rates of economic growth following the oil crisis of 1973, the continued rapid growth of health-care spending has led to urgent action in most countries to try to contain or reduce costs, the bulk of which fall in the public sector. Now that people in so many highly industrialized countries are working four or more weeks out of the year simply to pay for their health care, it is not surprising that more and more people are asking whether they are getting their money's worth from this vast expenditure.

One response to this reexamination of national priorities has been a desire to learn from the experiences of other countries. How does our health-care spending compare with that of others? Why do some countries spend more of their resources on health care than others? Have other countries found better answers to the questions of how to control costs, how to organize and finance health services so that resources are used efficiently, and how to establish priorities so that any extra resources bring the maximum gain in terms of health improvement? What are the long-term underlying forces leading to the escalation of health-care costs? Should these forces be moderated, checked, or controlled, and if so, how?

Questions of this kind cannot be sensibly approached without a hard body of fact describing and analyzing the present situation and the trends that have led to it on a strictly comparable international basis. Although most countries have by now developed series of figures analyzing trends in health-care expenditure for national purposes, there is still, as Maxwell points out, no internationally agreed-on definition of health care or of its component parts. As a result, the different figures obtainable from national sources are not strictly comparable. Maxwell makes a major contribution by specifying so many of these different causes of lack of comparability and identifying what is and what is not included in each of the series of national figures that he analyzes and attempts to compare.

Many of these problems could be resolved if there were an internationally agreed-on definition to which national statistical series were adjusted to conform. This would undoubtedly be a great step forward. But it would be wrong to assume that all the problems could be resolved in this way unless we were content to define health care as services provided and supervised by health-trained personnel and to look no further than that. It is inevitable that the social functions performed by health-trained personnel differ between countries and that the same type of need may be met by health-trained personnel in one country and by persons with social-welfare training or by family members in another. Maxwell is right to stress that the border between health care and social-welfare care is by far the most difficult to handle in cross-national comparisons.

The lack of strictly comparable data is not the only problem underlying international comparisons. Other problems arise when attempts are made to compare national data either using rates of exchange or in terms of proportions of GNP. The former are far from providing fair indicators of the purchasing power of national currencies. And comparisons in terms of GNP can be seriously misleading if those working in health care receive different relative earnings within their national economies.

Maxwell warns the reader of these and other limitations both in the data and in the method of analysis he is using. It is, however, very unlikely that all these causes of inadequate comparability seriously distort his main findings. He presses his analysis further than most earlier studies by attempting breakdowns of health-care expenditure both by type of service and by sources of funds. He also distinguishes carefully between the public financing of services and the public ownership of services. Overall, he presents the most comprehensive analysis of health-care spending that has so far been published.

Brian Abel-Smith
The London School of
Economics and Political Science

1 Introduction

This book is an attempt to document total health-care expenditures (public and private) for a cross-section of ten developed countries. It updates previous studies to 1977 or later—depending on the availability of data in each country—and for 1975 analyzes the composition of health-care expenditures in a standard format.

International studies of this type are fraught with difficulties. There is as yet no international machinery for the collection and analysis of health-care expenditure data. Not only is there no standard accounting format, but terms are not even agreed and defined.

Nevertheless, individual countries have shown rapidly growing interest in collecting data in this field. Governments and others concerned with meeting the bills, such as employers and trade unions, want to know what health services cost and how the money is spent. Health-care spending now represents up to one-tenth of total national expenditures and for some levels of government forms a much higher proportion of public expenditures. Moreover, in the 1960s and early 1970s health-care spending grew consistently faster than gross national product (GNP), raising increasingly uncomfortable questions about how further increases were to be financed. Particularly with a downturn in economic growth, more government money could be found for health care year after year only by cutting back other public programs or by increasing taxes. As a long-term solution neither alternative was attractive, and it was therefore inevitable that expenditure on health services should come under close scrutiny.

Therefore, countries such as the United States, France, and Canada now maintain and publish annual statistics on their health-care expenditures. From their statistical series they can, with certain reservations, tell how much was spent on health services in their own countries and how this compared with earlier years and with changes in prices and in GNP. Once they have this information and begin to ask sensible questions about it, the importance of international comparisons becomes apparent. Questions such as "Do we spend enough or too much?" "Do we have the right balance of expenditure?" and "Do we obtain good value for what we spend?" are natural ones to ask about health-care expenditures, but are nonetheless largely unanswerable. A constructive step toward answering them is to try first to answer questions such as "How do we compare with others in the amount that we spend, in our patterns of expenditure, and in the value that

1

we appear to receive?'' These questions call not only for national data but also for data from other countries in a comparable form and using similar definitions. To date, that information is for the most part lacking.

One can argue, of course, that aggregated information will in any event have little value, since it will merely illustrate that other countries are also spending large quantities of scarce resources on activities of unproved benefit. For this reason many health economists prefer at this stage to concentrate on micro analysis, whereby it should prove more possible to assess preferences, costs, results, and the interrelationships among them. But it is perhaps even more shortsighted to reject the case for any macro analysis than to ignore its limitations. If we pursue micro analysis alone, we will lose sight of the larger picture into which it must fit, yet that picture does exist and has some characteristics that we forget at our peril. Moreover, ministers of health, ministers of finance, and governments are inevitably concerned at least as much with the macro as with the micro level; and it seems appropriate to take macro analysis as far as its limitations will allow in order to help them in some of the decisions that they must make. Finally, in policy terms the broad trends are important, perhaps particularly when they appear to be common to many countries. International data are generally inconclusive as to why one country differs from others, and may do no more than suggest a line of further investigation. High pharmaceutical expenditures in West Germany and France are examples. But patterns that are similar across a range of countries, despite all the difficulties of comparison and the national differences, are unlikely to be misleading. The sustained growth in health-care expenditures in the 1960s and early 1970s at a faster rate than the growth of GNP was one example, and the swing from private to public financing was another. A change in those trends would also be of great importance for health-care policy.

Ultimately, however, arguments like these will not persuade the skeptics that a study such as this has much merit. Whatever its limits may be, there is value in clarifying the broad frame of financial reference into which we can fit more detailed information.

Earlier Studies of Health-Care Expenditures

The ancestry of the present study lies in part with national data series. Of these that of the United States is the oldest, providing annual estimates of health-care expenditures from all sources, private as well as public, in a coherent sequence from 1929 onward [1]. CREDOC (Centre de recherche pour l'étude et l'observation des conditions de vie) provides a regular expenditure series in France, with very careful definitions of what the figures contain, and also publishes much fuller analyses on selected topics, such as phar-

maceutical expenditures and regional differences [2]. Health and Welfare
Canada now issues regular health-care-expenditure reports for Canada
with a statistical series dating from 1960 [3]. Of the other countries included in the present study, Sweden, the United Kingdom, and the
Netherlands all publish government estimates covering at least the major
elements of national health-care expenditures, although these are not in as
convenient a form as those of the United States, France, and Canada. The
remaining four countries included are moving toward the establishment of
data series but are still heavily dependent on the efforts of a few individuals,
some of whom are mentioned specifically later in this introductory chapter.

It is relatively unusual for any of these data series to be cross-national,
although CREDOC has produced cross-national comparisons on selected
topics, and the Canadian series includes American figures. The earliest genuinely international study was *The Cost of Medical Care*, published by the
International Labor Office (ILO) in 1959 [4]. This study tackled the
almost superhuman task of comparing the medical-care payments provided
under social-security systems in fourteen countries with payments provided
under voluntary insurance in the United States. The figures presented span
the period 1945-1955. The authors encountered most of the problems
familiar to later researchers in this field, such as differences in currency
values, coverage, and definitions, and tackled them imaginatively. For example, all expenditures are expressed per person protected by each scheme,
in terms of (1) the average annual income per head in the country concerned, (2) the annual reference wage, and (3) the national income per
economically active person. Expenditures are not merely aggregated but
are, where possible, given separately for the main facets of health care, such
as physicians' services, pharmaceutical benefits, and hospital services.
Because entitlements varied so much from scheme to scheme, estimates also
had to be made (per person protected) for other payments by government
and by individuals. The cautious assumption was made that national differences in relative expenditure were likely to be wholly or largely results of
differences in the nature and extent of the benefits provided; in other
words, for the purposes of the study there were assumed to be no differences in costs relative to national income nor in cost effectiveness.
Despite the sweeping nature of this assumption, the conclusions reached by
this study were of great importance. The total cost of medical care per
person covered was found to vary relatively little (from around 1.75 to
around 2 percent of average national income at factor cost per economically
active person), regardless of the country or the method of providing medical
care. The main variations among countries appeared to result from differences in the cost of pharmaceuticals. Very tentatively it was inferred
from the cross-national comparisons that costs were highest in countries in
which there was direct access to specialist care. In contrast with some later

studies, and despite the widespread apprehension from which the study originated, medical-care expenditures by social-security organizations did not then appear to be rising appreciably faster than national income (except in France and Italy). The main danger was thought to lie in a further increase in hospital costs, particularly in the cost of maintaining and nursing the patient, rather than in the cost of medical treatment.

The next major initiative in this field was taken by the World Health Organization (WHO) and led in due course to two publications by Brian Abel-Smith. The first of these, *Paying for Health Services*, was a feasibility study conducted in six countries in order to establish a workable methodology for the study of health costs [5]. The six countries—Ceylon, Chile, Czechoslovakia, Israel, Sweden, and the United States—were deliberately selected to include varying systems for financing health services, as well as different standards of living. The questionnaire that was used was revised in light of the study to propose a standard classification for the recording of national expenditures on health services. Such a classification naturally required careful definition of both costs and services. *Costs* excluded loss of income and the payment of cash benefits, and included only the real resources used in providing health services. *Health services* were defined as all medical care given to individuals; public-health services, including preventive services and surveillance (but only the medical supervision of environmental services); and research and teaching, including medical education.

Current operating costs were divided into four groups: payments to personnel, payments for provisions, payments for pharmaceuticals and medical supplies, and payments for other goods and services. Depreciation, where charged, was excluded from current operating costs on the grounds that in many countries no such item was included in hospital accounts and that there were bound to be substantial differences in the method of computation. (However, one of the conclusions drawn from the study was that it would be preferable in future work to include within current costs rent, rates, depreciation on buildings and equipment calculated on a "straight-line" basis over a given number of years, and interest on capital employed.) Capital costs included land purchase; expenditure on new buildings and on the adaptation or extension of existing buildings; and the cost of initial furniture, equipment, and supplies for new and adapted buildings. (Again, some changes in these definitions were proposed in the study's conclusions.) The questionnaire and standard classification also covered sources of finance for health services, distinguishing between direct payment (made by the patient and not recovered by him from voluntary insurance) and indirect payment. Indirect payment was subdivided into general government funds, compulsory social insurance, voluntary insurance, and charitable and voluntary donations. All expenditures were related to gross national expenditure (GNE) in the country concerned.

(GNE differs from GNP in its inclusion of net transfers and borrowing from abroad. In most countries there is little difference between GNP and GNE; however, Israel, which was included in this study, was at that time a notable exception, with a 12.3 percent lower figure for GNP than for GNE.)

The data produced in this first WHO report could be compared cross-nationally only with great caution, in view of the deliberately diverse selection of countries and the different accounting years used by them. Data were for only one accounting year for each country, and the years varied between calendar 1956 and the twelve months ending 31 March 1960. Indeed, the data were essentially illustrative and the principal conclusions were methodological. The standard accounting classification proposed has been a common point of reference ever since and has influenced the development of a language of health-service finance, although unfortunately it has not yet led to the adoption of a uniform system in national accounts.

The second WHO report, also by Brian Abel-Smith, was *An International Study of Health Expenditure*, published in 1967 [6]. It stemmed directly from the methodological work described in the first report, using the classifications developed in it and extending the analysis to twenty-nine countries. The objectives were to compile comparable international information about expenditure on health services and their component parts, as well as on financing methods, and to develop a standardized framework for national-health accounting.

In some respects the data demands made on countries participating in the main study proved to be too great. For example, the feasibility report's breakdown of current operating costs into four categories of payments (personnel, provisions, pharmaceuticals, and other goods and services) was replaced in the main study by a breakdown into sixteen categories. Few countries were able to provide a complete or even nearly complete return in such detail. In addition they were asked to show separately and to include in their total health-care expenditures such items as imputed rent, interest, and depreciation. Only three of the twenty-nine countries gave separate figures for depreciation, and only two made any return for imputed rent. Accordingly, both depreciation and rent were excluded, wherever practicable, from the cross-national comparisons.

More important inconsistencies among countries were differences in their definitions of environmental services and the regulatory activities relating to them. Some countries, such as Venezuela, used a far broader definition than others. Medications posed another problem, especially since the twenty-nine countries spanned widely different cultures and stages of development. A tribal remedy used in Senegal might not be classified as a medicinal drug in Sweden, nor was the range of medications necessarily the same even in countries of similar levels of wealth. To determine direct expenditure by recipients of services, most countries made estimates based on consumer surveys and other sources. Such estimates were subject to substantial variations of definition and to wide margins of error.

Nevertheless, the figures for total health-care expenditures, which were mainly for 1961, were thought to be broadly comparable. For all but four of the countries making full returns, the error was thought to lie in the range of ±5 percent. The remaining four might, it was thought, have an error of ±15 percent. Countries not making full returns frequently could not estimate direct expenditures by patients, but in most cases their estimates of indirect expenditures by third parties were relatively complete.

The resulting data were related for each country to GNP and to national income (net national product at factor cost, excluding depreciation allowances, subsidies, and taxes). Total expenditure on health services, including capital, in 1961 or the nearest available year, fell in the range of 2.5-6.3 percent of GNP, with most developed countries exceeding 4 percent. Cautious use was also made of comparisons in U.S. dollars per head at current rates of exchange. Capital expenditure was related to gross domestic capital formation. Percentage breakdowns of total expenditures were calculated, by financing source and by main service, for example. Attempts were made to assess expenditure patterns and trends and to identify explanatory variables.

Some of the findings were negative in that there appeared to be no coherent pattern. But at least two important conclusions were drawn. First, it was concluded that the "healthiest" countries (judged in terms of mortality) spent most on health services, rather than those countries that, by this criterion, seemed in greatest need of high expenditure. Second, it was perceived that in all high-income countries except the United Kingdom there had been (in the 1950s) a secular trend for expenditure on health services to increase as a proportion of national income or national product. This rate of increase was such that an additional 1 percent of GNP was likely to be absorbed in health services every ten years. If this trend continued, before the end of the century some countries would be devoting more than 10 percent of GNP to health care. Both these conclusions have been widely accepted and have had substantial influence across the broad fields of health economics and health-policy analysis. In addition, the data provided by the study have been extensively used in other work, in default of other internationally comparable figures for health-care expenditures.

In December 1970 and again in March 1973, J.G. Simanis published in the *Social Security Bulletin* updated estimates that he hoped were comparable with those in the Abel-Smith study [7]. The 1973 article contained estimates of 1969 health-care expenditures as a percentage of GNP for Canada, France, West Germany, the Netherlands, Sweden, the United Kingdom, and the United States. The estimates ranged from 4.8 percent in the United Kingdom to 7.3 percent in Canada. These figures were not obtained by conducting another cross-national survey but by selecting and weighting available statistics that had in combination approximated the level of expenditures reported in the WHO study. Rates of increase were also calculated for health-care expenditures from the differences between the WHO figures and the updated estimates; and these were compared with changes in other economic indicators, such as the consumer price and wage indexes and GNP. Overall, it appeared that health-care spending had risen even faster in the 1960s than in the 1950s: Whereas the increase in the 1950s was of the order of 1 percent of GNP, in the 1960s it seemed likely to exceed 1.5 percent in most of the countries included.

Another major study in this field, with a somewhat different emphasis, was undertaken by the Organization for Economic Cooperation and Development (OECD), resulting in the publication in 1977 of *Public Expenditure on Health* [8]. This was part of a broad, continuing review by OECD of public-expenditure trends in member countries. In the early 1970s OECD's Economic Policy Committee began to take a keen interest in questions of resource allocation and the choices open to governments. Reports were published on education, income maintenance, and then health, as part of a series on major public-expenditure programs. Data for the health study were provided by twenty-four member governments for 1974 and 1962 (or the nearest available years) and were printed in a lengthy annex to the report. The report is carefully documented and is imaginative in its use of explanatory factors and statistical techniques. Expenditures were related to "trend" gross domestic product (GDP), which differs from GNP through the exclusion of net income from abroad. Trend GDP was calculated by the use of deflators developed by OECD. For 1974 the OECD average for total health-care spending (excluding capital expenditure) was 5.7 percent of GDP, of which public spending accounted for 4.4 percent. The latter figure had increased from 2.5 percent in the early 1960s.

The main emphasis throughout is on *public* expenditure, since this is the focus of OECD concern. Public health-care expenditures were broken down by main source of finance and by major service: hospitals, ambulatory medical services, medical supplies, and other. Reasons for intercountry differences in public-sector spending on health care were sought in terms of a use ratio (particularly hospital days per person covered), a coverage ratio (the proportion of the population covered by public health insurance), a transfer ratio (the proportion of total cost met directly or indirectly by the public sector), and a cost ratio. The last of these was, in concept, a measure of the unit cost of health care in the country concerned in terms of its GDP per capita. One of the most interesting comparisons made, which will be discussed later in this chapter, was of doctors' income in relation to GDP per capita and earned income; but definitions of income were inconsistent, and the differences could not in any case be used in estimating the cost ratio because of the lack of other relevant data. In practice, for the main cross-national comparisons, the cost ratio had to be estimated as a residual.

These same ratios were used to assess why, between 1962 and 1974, public expenditure on health services had increased relative to GDP. Changes in utilization and in relative prices appeared to be the principal causes, but the authors were not entirely convinced of the validity of this conclusion. They saw two possible future scenarios. In one, public expenditure on health services would continue to increase relative to GDP, but at a somewhat slower rate. In the other, which the report appears to favor, governments would make a determined and successful bid to stabilize public-sector spending on health care in terms of GDP. Possible lines for government action were suggested, including the transfer back to users of a larger share of expenditure; tighter controls over utilization and supply; substitution of less-expensive labor; and reductions in fees for medical services and in pharmaceutical prices.

More recent international estimates of health-care expenditures include a 1978 report to the European Commission by Abel-Smith and Maynard [9]; a short section in another 1978 European Commission report by Abel-Smith and Grandjeat on pharmaceutical consumption [10]; and a 1979 survey by Hauser and Koch of the Saint Gall Graduate School of Economics, Switzerland, for an international seminar on health-care costs [11]. Each of these studies encountered the familiar problems of lack of comparable data. Abel-Smith and Maynard used various national estimates, noting briefly what these estimates comprised. Current costs of health services are given relative to GNP for nine countries for the period 1966-1975, with 1976 data for a few countries. The main emphasis is on common trends shown by the national series rather than on international differences, in view of lack of cross-national comparability of definitions.

Abel-Smith and Grandjeat [10] concentrate on the cross-national comparison of pharmaceutical consumption, and we will return to their study in that context. They found themselves having to make estimates of total health-care expenditures in order to put pharmaceutical expenditure in context, but they did not place much reliance on the overall expenditure figures. Hauser and Koch [11] had neither the time nor the resources to undertake an in-depth study and therefore used a questionnaire that was answered by selected seminar participants. Their findings principally concern the proportional structure of finance (where the money comes from) and expenditure (the health services on which it is spent) within countries, and changes in these proportions between 1960 and 1975.

Thus up to now there have been only four major international studies of health expenditures: the ILO study of the period 1945-1955; the two linked WHO studies by Brian Abel-Smith, concentrating on the 1950s and culminating in an extensive cross-national comparison for 1961; and, finally, the OECD study, which focuses on public expenditure in 1962 and 1974, with relatively little attention given to private-sector spending.

Other Relevant Studies

There have, of course, been many other studies with an international dimension. Good work has been done on international variations in pharmaceutical pricing [12], prescribing patterns [13], and pharmaceutical expenditures [14]. W.A. Glaser has compared methods of paying doctors [15] and, more generally, mechanisms used in different countries for setting fees and controlling costs under health-insurance plans [16]. A start has been made on looking at international differences in patterns of medical treatment [17], although in this field the surface has barely been scratched. In the last ten years descriptions have been published of health systems in most countries, with broad comparisons among groups with similar systems or at similar stages of economic development [18]. There has also been a great expansion of writing on health economics [19], as well as some important, seminal work on epidemiology and health strategy [20].

A final category of work that deserves mention in connection with the present study is analysis of the relationships among national wealth, health-care expenditures, and health needs. Although the early studies were national in focus, they might well have been international had the necessary data been available. It is natural that some of the earliest commentaries were British, in view of public debate about the cost of the National Health Service. As early as 1952 Dr. Ffrangcon Roberts wrote a brilliant short book, *The Cost of Health* [21]. Some of its comments were far in advance of its time and have freshness and resonance even now. Costs for the National Health Service had been vastly underestimated before it was set up. By 1952 expenditure was already well over twice the level that Beveridge had predicted as a plateau lasting until 1965. Why was this so? Dr. Roberts suggested four possible answers, of which the most perceptive is that the advance of medicine may paradoxically increase the true incidence of disease. The further medicine advances, the greater is the amount of work that it makes for itself, because more of the young then survive to join the old and to suffer diseases that are much more difficult to cure. The health professions, like Sisyphus, will never succeed in pushing this stone to the top of the slope. Meanwhile, medicine may make vast scientific strides, since the possibilities for greater knowledge are virtually unlimited. We are therefore face to face with the paradox of potentially unlimited progress towards an unattainable objective. As time passes, what is practically possible will fall further and further short of what is theoretically feasible. The resources available will never be sufficient; indeed, they will become increasingly inadequate. The medical profession and health-care administrators will have to decide how to put limited resources to best use. "The expense of the health service is incurred by individuals acting singly; the bill is paid by individuals acting collectively. There is therefore a permanent conflict between the demand for greater expenditure and the demand for smaller expenditure, a conflict which is present in the mind of almost every individual, although he may be quite unconscious of its existence" [22]. A national health service is only feasible if individuals exercise restraint and identify their fellows' interests with their own.

Another British doctor, J.R. Seale, published articles in the *Lancet* in 1959 and 1960 [23]. In the second of these he applied the management-accounting concept of fixed and variable costs to health services. Most of the costs of health services were fixed, he argued, and were little altered by changes in use. The first, and more important, article stated a general theory of national expenditure on medical care. He used the U.S. data series from 1929 to illustrate his theory that the proportion of GNP devoted to medical care by any nation tended in the long run to remain constant. The percentage rose during national economic depressions (particularly in the Great Depression of the 1930s, but also in the period immediately following the Korean War), and it fell during wars. A persistent rise in real per-capita GNP would tend to result in a very gradual increase in health-care spending relative to GNP.

Although the 1960s were to be a decade of much faster increases in health-care expenditure than Seale's general theory predicted, the evidence supporting the theory remains strong for the twenty-five years up to the mid-1950s. A revised general theory would therefore still have to take account of this evidence, as well as of what has happened since.

The ILO study previously mentioned [4] was published at much the same time as Seale's *Lancet* articles, and the WHO reports by Abel-Smith [5, 6] followed in 1963 and 1967. These provided further stimulus to thinking about macroeconomic issues in health-care policy, as well as data that were extensively quoted. The broad conclusions of the 1967 report about the growth of health-care expenditures and the lack of correlation between expenditures and needs were generally accepted. Rising concern (particularly by governments) about the steep expenditure increases of the 1960s and early 1970s was reflected not only in the OECD study *Public Expenditure on Health* [8] but also in international seminars and the publications resulting from them [24]. The latter were valuable less for the data they contained than as a means of exchanging views about their implications.

By the mid-1970s commentary on these issues had become so widespread that any brief description of the literature is likely to be idiosyncratic. Among the most interesting were articles by H.H. Hiatt in 1974,

J.P. Newhouse in 1976, and A.L. Cochrane and others in 1978. Howard Hiatt, in *Protecting the Medical Commons: Who is Responsible?* [25], drew on Garrett Hardin's concept of the tragedy of the commons. There had to be a limit to the resources any society could devote to health care, just as there was a limit to the grazing area on the commons; and the United States might, Hiatt contended, be approaching that limit. If so, it was high time for thought to be given to the best use of those resources. Otherwise, urgent additional demands, such as those to address the current inadequacy of medical care for large sectors of the population, could not be accommodated (as they ought to be) on the "commons."

Brian Abel-Smith had pointed to the lack of correspondence between health needs and health-care expenditure [6]. In fact, by what Julian Tudor-Hart came to enunciate as the Inverse Care Law [26], expenditure appears to be least where the need is greatest. J.P. Newhouse of the Rand Corporation, in an article in the *Journal of Human Resources* in 1976, elegantly stated the corollary to this [27]. If need does not determine health-care spending, what does? The answer is implicit in Abel-Smith's second report but is not explicitly stated there [6]. Newhouse filled the gap by demonstrating that 90 percent of the variance in per-capita medical-care expenditure for thirteen developed countries could be explained by variation in per-capita GDP. It would follow that no other variable (such as differences in the health-care delivery system) would be likely to make much difference.

Undeterred by conventional wisdom that national health status cannot be reliably assessed or compared by present measures, Cochrane, St. Leger, and Moore analyzed health-care "inputs" and health-status "outputs" for eighteen developed countries [28]. Inputs comprised health-service indexes (such as doctors, nurses, and acute-care hospital beds per 10,000 population; and percentage of GNP spent on health care); dietary indexes (including cigarette smoking, alcohol consumption, and caloric intake); and economic and demographic factors (population density, GNP per head, and the extent to which health-care expenditure was publicly rather than privately financed). Outputs were expressed in terms of age-specific mortality rates up to the age of 64. The article is an attractive mixture of careful statistical analysis, gentle irony, and seriousness. GNP per head and (more surprisingly) population density, sugar consumption, and the extent of public financing of health care were all negatively correlated with mortality rates; thus they appeared to be "good" for health status in varying degrees for the different age groups. The "bad" inputs were cigarette smoking, alcohol consumption, and, embarrassingly, the ratio of doctors to population. No other indicator of health-service provision appeared to have much importance, either positive or negative, in explaining differences in mortality. This perhaps is a suitable cautionary note on which to end a review of previous international studies.

The Present Study

The present study had three objectives. The first was simply to provide reasonably reliable and comparable information about health-care expenditures for a cross section of developed countries up to the most recent date possible. The second goal, if the framework of the analysis proved sound, was to propose a structure for future national and international data collection. Additionally, it was hoped that some conclusions, however tentative, could be drawn for health policy.

In concept the study is closest to the Abel-Smith study for WHO, and particularly to Abel-Smith's 1967 report, *An International Study of Health Expenditure* [6], in that it concentrates first on data collection and is concerned with health-care spending from *all* sources. In making cross-national comparisons of health and health services in the mid-1970s [29], the lack of data about health-care expenditures was both striking and surprising. Data were regularly published by WHO on population, mortality, infectious morbidity, and such key health-care resources as medical and nursing manpower and hospital beds. But expenditures, which were of great interest to analysts and to governments, were not available through WHO for any date later than 1961 (the base year for the Abel-Smith study). This study is an attempt to fill the gap.

The ten countries included in the study are Australia, Canada, France, West Germany, Italy, the Netherlands, Sweden, Switzerland, the United Kingdom, and the United States. Developing countries were excluded since the nature of their health-care problems and the scale of their resources are so utterly different that they call for a separate study. So does the communist bloc, with its very different national-accounting conventions. The criteria used in selecting among Western, developed countries were population size (small nations were, in general, excluded); familiarity (hence Japan had to be excluded because I did not feel able to interpret any statistical information received); and particular interest (thus Sweden, the Netherlands, and Switzerland all have a health-care-systems importance beyond their population size).

This last point requires some elaboration. Sweden was included because it has one of the most advanced and expensive systems of health-care provision in the world. An international study of health services that excluded Sweden would be like a tennis tournament without the game's leading player. Switzerland's health system is much less well known but is notable for its strongly decentralized and diverse nature, as well as for the high standards of health care. The Netherlands similarly has much local variety, although it differs from Switzerland in having unitary government rather than cantonal governments in a loose federation. The Netherlands also has exceptionally well-developed arrangements for health care in the community, including care of the elderly and the handicapped. In systems characteristics it stands somewhere between the Scandinavian and British systems on the one hand and those of Germany and France on the other.

Total health-care spending was determined for each country for 1950, 1955, 1960, 1965, 1970, and as many of the succeeding years as possible. Partly as a check on the comparability and internal consistency of the totals, and partly in search of patterns within totals, a standard breakdown of health-care expenditures was required for each country for 1974 and 1975 or the nearest available years. The standard breakdown of the total was in four parts, each representing a different perspective on expenditures:

1. *Sources of finance*: Where does the money come from to pay for health care?
2. *Control of the supply side*: Who owns and administers the institutions and services through which health care is delivered?
3. *Resources used*: What resources of manpower and supplies does the money buy for use in health care?
4. *Services provided*: What health services are provided? (One immediately wants to add "to whom, and with what result?" but that question is, for the present, beyond reach of any but the most rudimentary answers on an international basis.)

There is, of course, a complex interrelationship among these four. Money from various public and private sources flows through a variety of public and private institutions and agencies, to pay people and buy supplies, so that services can be delivered. Some of the variations are missed by looking at each perspective in turn—for example, whether publicly administered institutions differ substantially from private ones in their pattern of resource use or in the services that they provide. Nevertheless, one must start somewhere, and it is probably better to start simply.

The method used was to prepare a standard chart of accounts for each of these four expenditure perspectives, with a list of questions on definitions. Next, an expert individual or group in each country, who could help to fill in the chart of accounts for the selected years and answer the questions, was approached. People had to be found who understood the purposes of the study and knew their own national data sources well. By this means it was possible to shorten enormously the task of data collection and interpretation. Sometimes the choice was obvious, as with CREDOC in France and the Health Care Financing Administration of the Department of Health, Education and Welfare (DHEW), now the Department of Health and Human Services, in the United States. In other cases it was far more difficult. Those who provided this invaluable help, and to whom I am profoundly grateful, are

Australia: Dr. John Deeble, Australian National University, Canberra and Alan Mackay, Policy and Planning Division, Commonwealth Department of Health, Canberra.

Canada: William A. Mennie, director, Health Economics and Data Analysis, Health and Welfare Canada, Ottawa.

France: Madame Simone Sandier and Marc Duriez, CREDOC, Paris.

Germany: Dr. H. Essig and Herr W. Müller at Statistisches Bundesamt, Wiesbaden.

Italy: Professor Antonio Brenna and Dr. Vittorio Mapelli, Istituto per la ricerca di Economia Sanitaria, Milan.

Netherlands: Dr. Frans Rutten, Ministerie van Volksgezondheid en Milieuhygiene, The Hague.

Sweden: Dr. Gunnar Wennström, Socialstyrelsen; and Jan Redeby and Jörgen Enmark, Statistiska Centralbyrån, Stockholm.

Switzerland: Dr. Pierre Gygi, Wirtschaftstudien, Bern.

United States: Robert M. Gibson, Health Care Financing Administration, Department of Health and Human Services, Washington, D.C.

The figures could not have been compiled without their aid; the responsibility for errors lies, naturally, with me. Similarly, Professor Brian Abel-Smith was unstinting in his wise guidance. I also owe a great debt to the Sandoz Institute in Geneva, which funded this study, and to its staff Raymond Rigoni, Philip Selby, and Adrian Griffiths, for their encouragement and advice. Dr. Archie Cochrane contributed his characteristic enthusiasm, and Sir George Godber his equally characteristic firm support. Finally, my thanks to those at St. Thomas' Hospital, London, who have helped me in various ways: Johannes Goldschmidt for aid with statistics and computing; Professor Walter Holland for his contacts; the staff of the Special Trustees' office for typing and for patience beyond the call of duty; and the Special Trustees themselves.

Compared with earlier work, the main claim for the present study is one of updating. True, the updating is by only a few years with respect to the OECD study. But the two are not in competition. OECD was concerned very largely with public expenditures. The present study is broader in scope, although less sophisticated, and takes less for granted in terms of the underlying data. The Abel-Smith reports for WHO are a much closer model for the present study, and with respect to those reports the updating is by more than a decade. The chart of accounts and definitions used in the present study have many similarities to Abel-Smith's, although they were not directly modeled on his. The accounting framework is perhaps a little neater in its recognition of the four facets of health-care expenditures, each adding up to a total that reconciles with that for the other three facets. The search for a model for future data collection echoes his—much of the drudgery entailed would not have been required if his recommendations for the recording of national health-care expenditures had been implemented. Conclusions drawn for health policy are naturally different from his, since the context has changed.

The core of the present study is the national charts of accounts and the accompanying notes, which will be found in appendix C. From them are derived the summary tables in the text and the figures based on them. For ease of reading, data sources, definitions, and qualifications are not repeated in the main body of the text but can all be found in the national sections. The text itself deals with four broad areas: chapter 2 is concerned with methodology; chapter 3 describes overall trends in health-care expenditures; chapter 4 discusses the composition of these expenditures in terms of sources of funds and patterns of spending; and chapter 5 contains conclusions and implications.

2 Methods, Sources, and Definitions

A detailed description of the course of the study would be tedious. But a brief description is necessary in order to alert readers to the qualifications that must apply to the results. These qualifications are not lessened by a recognition that they would probably be inevitable in any similar international study of this subject at this time.

There are, of course, problems of data availability and reliability. No individual who was undertaking this type of research could set up his own independent data-collection system to record in ten different countries the costs of health-care transactions accounting for up to one-tenth of each nation's disposable wealth. One is forced to piece together from various sources information that has already been recorded for other purposes or that can be reliably estimated. This involves facing major questions of comparability and therefore of definition. What is included within, or excluded from, the expenditure recorded by a particular data source?

Process of the Study

The approach taken for the present study was first to design a standard chart of accounts reflecting a number of assumptions about the definition of health-care expenditures, and then to try to complete it for each of the ten countries for 1974 and 1975. The blank chart of accounts is attached as appendix A. It is accompanied by a list of questions that were used to assess the comparability of the data for that country with the corresponding entries for the other countries. The underlying assumptions about definitions are discussed later in this chapter.

In nearly all countries the sequence of research steps was the same. First, an expert was identified and asked to help in the study. Sometimes this was someone I already knew well, like Madame Simone Sandier at CREDOC in Paris, or Professor Antonio Brenna, director of the Istituto per la ricerca di Economia Sanitaria in Milan. More often it was someone whose work I knew, either as a researcher in this field or as a senior government official concerned with health-services statistics. In several cases the individual who had been approached introduced me to someone else who was in a better position to help. Occasionally, as in West Germany and Sweden, the search for an appropriate person proved a long one. A letter was then written to the individual concerned, explaining the purpose of the study and enclosing the chart of accounts and list of questions. At the same time a visit was arranged to take place soon after the arrival of the papers, so that I could either complete the chart of accounts under his supervision or check through his draft entries. Back-up calculations and references were recorded, and answers to the questions on the checklist were obtained. Usually some substantial further work was required in order to extract or estimate additional data from less-immediately accessible sources. Having returned to London with the data and received any later additions and revisions, I checked for inconsistencies with the sources, for internal anomalies, and for figures that seemed improbable by comparison with those for other countries. A further process of joint checking and revision followed, until the information appeared as complete and reliable as possible. The product at this stage was the national data summary for the country concerned, with its accompanying footnotes. These appear in appendix C.

The main exceptions were Canada, the United States, and the United Kingdom. Primarily for cost reasons, it was not possible to visit North America and collect the data on the spot. W.A. Mennie and his colleagues in the Health Economics and Data Analysis Division of Health and Welfare Canada went to great trouble to handle the data collection and its checking and revision at a distance. For the United States the data published by the U.S. Department of Health and Human Services is more complete and more fully explained than for any other country (except perhaps France). I had to rely essentially on this single source with some supplementing and guidance by Robert M. Gibson, who has recently been responsible for its compilation. For the United Kingdom I used a variety of statistical sources, mainly government publications, as recorded in the footnotes to the national summary. For manpower costs for the National Health Service, which have not recently been published in the necessary form, J.W. Hurst of the Economic Adviser's Office at the Department of Health and Social Security was extremely helpful.

When the national summaries were available, international tables were prepared from them. The final versions of these, with their accompanying footnotes, appear at the appropriate points in chapters 3 to 5 of this book. The last step was to write up the results, incorporating later information when it became available.

Starting Assumptions on Definitions

The standard chart of accounts (see appendix A) has four main sections comprising the sources of health-care finance, the mix of organizations through which it is spent, the health services provided, and the resources used.

The third of these sections assumed that health services comprise the following (for the whole population, including the armed forces and all other specific groups):

1. hospital and similar institutional medical services, whether provided on an inpatient or ambulatory basis;
2. primary and specialist health care outside hospitals;
3. self-care (which in practice proved to be the cost of self-medication or of drugs purchased without prescription);
4. public-health services (including immunization and other preventive activities, health education, and the medical supervision of environmental services);
5. medical and health-services research;
6. training of health-services personnel;
7. administration of all these services.

Capital expenditure was to be included but shown separately for hospital services and for services outside the hospital. Notional charges of capital against running costs, such as amortization and depreciation, were to be deducted from running costs to avoid double counting. Social-welfare services were excluded, as were cash benefits except to the extent that these were used to pay for health services. Consequential costs borne by families and the community as a result of ill health, such as waiting time and lost earnings, were also excluded.

This is a reasonably comprehensive and noncontroversial definition of health services, similar to that used by Abel-Smith in the two WHO studies [5, 6]. But there are nevertheless problems within it.

The first section of the chart of accounts was intended for recording how these services were funded. The main divisions are between public finance; payments by consumers; and payments by others, such as charities and voluntary organizations. Within public finance, the principal breakdown is between funding from general taxation and that from compulsory insurance or social security. Under payments by consumers are included private, voluntary insurance, and charges that consumers are unable to recover from any third party. Similar definitions have been used in previous international studies [4, 5, 6, 8].

Section 2 of the chart of accounts has no exact parallel in previous international studies, although something like it has been used in national studies in Australia, Germany, and Switzerland. It sought to examine the mix of public and private organizations through which health services are delivered. The breakdown has three main parts: government institutions, owned and run by the state; nongovernment institutions, not run for profit, such as voluntary hospitals and charities; and private, for-profit institutions, contractors, and practitioners.

The last of the four sections was concerned with health-care spending by resource category. Manpower, the largest category, was broken down by occupational group, among doctors (general-practice and specialist); dentists; nurses (qualified and other); professional and technical staff; and administrative, clerical, and auxiliary staff. The second category, pharmaceuticals, was subdivided between prescribed and nonprescribed. Equipment and supplies was meant to cover the purchase, repair, and maintenance of equipment, as well as supply items, whether medical or nonmedical. The fourth category, buildings, was intended to include expenditure on new buildings and on the adaptation and repair of existing buildings (excluding work carried out by personnel directly employed, since this would appear under manpower). "Other" was the final, residual category of resource expenditure.

Besides seeking to determine expenditure on manpower, the study requested staffing numbers for the main occupational groups, in terms of whole-time equivalents (in other words, figures for part-time staff were to be adjusted).

The resource breakdown was more extensive than that in Professor Abel-Smith's first WHO study [5], in which there were four categories: personnel, provisions, pharmaceuticals and medical supplies, and other goods and services. For manpower the breakdown was somewhat more complete than that in his second WHO study [6], but for nonpersonnel items (where he had difficulty in practice in completing his questionnaire) it was substantially less detailed.

It was always intended in the present study that the chart of accounts should provide some internal checks, and these in fact proved useful. Each of the four sections had to add to the same total. If one did not, there must be a mathematical error or inconsistency of definition. Moreover, a major anomaly in comparisons between countries was likely to be much more obvious in one section of the analysis than in others.

Total health-care expenditure for the year in question was to be related to population and to gross national product (GNP) at market prices. The latter seemed the simplest measure of relative national income and the one most likely to be readily available.

Applying the Definitions in Practice

Table 2-1 summarizes the principal problems of definition that emerged in practice, and the extent to which there were variations among countries. In such matters as cash benefits, consequential costs imposed by illness, preventive activities and health education, and services given on a charitable basis, there appeared to be reasonable conformity to the standard definition. On two major matters—the boundary between hospital and other health-care costs, and the treatment of capital construction—there were very important differences, but ones that affected classifications within health-care expenditures rather than totals. For all the other items there were variations that did affect totals. However, since most items do not by themselves form a large proportion of total health-care expenditures, even a marked difference of definition of one item would not have a big impact on the total. Moreover, provided that a country was not consistently "high" or "low" on each definition, the differences would tend to balance one another. The most difficult single problem is likely to be the boundary with social welfare in the care of the elderly and handicapped, since the differences here could be large. For example the importance of nursing homes, and their classification, varies from country to country.

Overall, as shown at the foot of table 2-1, the totals for four countries appear low relative to others, owing to definitional problems. The difference is hard to quantify, but I would estimate the relative understatement as 5 to 10 percent for Switzerland and under 5 percent for Australia, Italy, and the Netherlands.

It is tempting to adjust the figures to make them seem more comparable, for example by adding a figure for over-the-counter (OTC) drugs in the Netherlands, or for ambulance costs in Switzerland. This was not done for two reasons. First, it seemed better to use for each country data that can be supported from its own statistical sources. Second, once one begins making adjustments, it is hard to know where to stop. Any remaining differences may merely reflect one's starting prejudices. Therefore, the results are not adjusted for the possible differences in definition, although I will assess in certain cases the effect of making such adjustments.

GNP at market prices was not available for Australia nor (from 1975 onward) for France. On the other hand, gross domestic product (GDP) was not uniformly available either. GNP at market prices was therefore used as the standard measure and was estimated from GDP when necessary. The year used for recording (calendar year or some other twelve-month period) varied. Australia, the United Kingdom, and the United States do not use the calendar year for their health-care-expenditure accounts. For certain of the comparisons, the figures for these countries were adjusted to a calendar-year basis; the variations are in all cases noted. Taxes on expenditure, such as value-added taxes and sales taxes, are not standard. Neither GNP nor health-care expenditures are adjusted for these differences. As far as health-care expenditures are concerned, the principal variations in these taxes are noted in line 17 of table 2-1.

In chapter 5 we will return to conclusions about data availability, reliability, and comparability, and about continuing data collection. Meanwhile it must be borne in mind that there are substantial difficulties inherent in such comparisons. I do not believe, however, that these difficulties invalidate the main findings.

Table 2-1
Definitions, Known Variations, and Additional Notes
(✓ indicates that country conforms to standard definition)

General Position (Standard Definition)	Australia	Canada	France	West Germany
1. *Coverage*: Health Services are intended to be included for the whole population, including the armed forces, the police, prisoners, transport workers, and industrial workers.	A relatively small amount of industrial medicine (for example, mining companies) is excluded.	Health services for forces overseas are excluded and, within Canada, the salaries of service personnel providing health care outside institutions.	✓	Services for the armed forces and for prisoners are largely excluded.
2. *Cash benefits*: All cash benefits are excluded, but reimbursement to patients for medical expenses paid are included	✓	✓	✓	✓
3. *Boundary with social welfare*: The boundary depends in practice on convention in the country concerned. Institutions and services of a predominantly medical nature (all hospitals, all physicians' fees, all services reimbursed under health insurance) are included. Residential homes and services for the aged and handicapped are excluded except where they are of a predominantly medical nature. At the margin there are variations among countries depending particularly on whether or not a hospital or other recognized health agency provides the service.	Criterion of "curative or palliative intent" applied and attempt made to exclude costs of services not meeting the criterion, such as care of the mentally handicapped and residential care of the elderly not undergoing medical treatment. Definition thus more restrictive than in Canada or the United States.	Definition of health-care expenditures a rather broad one, including nursing homes; homes for the aged; convalescent homes; and residential homes for the mentally ill, mentally handicapped, alcoholics, and drug addicts. On the other hand, some community services for these groups are excluded when not provided by hospitals or public-health agencies.	Costs of spa treatment are included, but represent only 0.5 percent of total costs. Hospitals and other institutions and services of a predominantly medical type are included. Nonmedical (such as homes for the elderly and handicapped) are generally excluded.	Costs of spa treatment are included and are substantial (5 percent of total health costs). The boundary between health and welfare depends, as in France, on the classification of the providing institution and whether the service concerned is funded under a health program (such as a health law).
4. *Boundary with education*: Education and training costs are included for training on the job in a health agency. The preclinical education of doctors and other university graduates is excluded except where noted. Nursing education is only excluded where provided through universities or colleges, rather than through health agencies.	Only one preclinical year excluded for medical students. Nursing education included.	Education and training costs excluded, except for further training provided to employees by health agencies. Nursing education, which is mainly provided in community colleges, is largely excluded.	Preclinical medical education is included, as is nursing education.	As in the standard definition. Nursing education is included.
5. *Boundary with environmental services*: Only medical supervision and surveillance of these services are included.	✓	✓	✓	✓
6. *Sundry services to patients*: The costs of education for children, of religious services (to the extent not met by the religions concerned), and of social work are included when provided within health-care institutions, but not otherwise. Domestic help at home is excluded. Cash allowances to hospital residents are excluded.	Education costs for children are thought to be excluded.	Costs of religious services largely excluded. Domestic help at home included when part of a home-care scheme approved by government.	These costs are mainly excluded.	✓

Italy	Netherlands	Sweden	Switzerland	United Kingdom	United States
✔	✔	Some private employers provide industrial-health services at their own cost, and these costs are excluded.	✔	Similar to Sweden.	✔
✔	✔	✔	✔	✔	✔
Services for alcoholics and drug addicts are largely classified as social expenditure rather than health-care. Similarly for the mentally and physically handicapped.	Definition of health-care expenditures includes nursing homes, homes for the mentally handicapped, services for alcoholics and drug addicts, and community services such as social psychiatric services and the preventive activities of the "cross" associations.	Institutions not providing a *medical* service tend to be excluded since they are run by local government, not by the county councils.	All nonmedical institutions are excluded except for payments to visiting physicians. Definition thus relatively restrictive.	All services under medical supervision are included, including services for the mentally and physically handicapped and for addicts. Residential homes for the elderly are excluded, as are private nursing homes for the elderly unless covered by health insurance.	To qualify as health-care institutions, nursing homes must have *at least half* their residents receiving nursing care. Thus up to half are not receiving nursing care, yet are included in health-care costs.
Similar to Germany.	As in the standard definition. Nursing education is increasingly being provided in separate colleges and is then excluded.	Similar to Canada.	Similar to Germany.	Similar to Germany.	Similar to Canada.
✔	✔	✔	✔	✔	✔
Education costs for children are thought to be excluded.	Social work and domestic help at home included when provided as part of the public system.	These costs are mainly excluded, except for medical social work in hospitals.	✔	✔	These costs are mainly excluded.

Table 2-1 *(continued)*

General Position *(Standard Definition)*	Australia	Canada	France	West Germany
7. *Charitable services*: Services are valued at cost and thus not included to the extent that they are provided free or below the market rate. The extent of understatement is relatively small.	✔	✔	✔	✔
8. *Prevention and health education*: These costs are included to the extent that the activities are undertaken under a health program. Immunization and infant and school health programs are all common. Health education is variable, but growing.	✔	✔	✔	✔
9. *Self-care*: Only the costs of self-medication (nonprescribed drugs) are included.	✔	✔	✔	✔
10. *Consequential costs*: Costs imposed on individuals and the community by ill health, such as lost earnings and waiting time, are excluded (see also item 2).	✔	✔	✔	✔
11. *Boundary between hospital and other health-care costs*: The practice varies, as noted, in two important ways: (1) fees paid to private physicians may be recorded in hospital costs or excluded from them; (2) hospital-based ambulatory care may be included or excluded from hospital costs. (Note that this problem does not affect total costs.)	Hospital costs exclude private fees. They include hospital-based ambulatory care.	Hospital costs include both items.	Hospital costs exclude both items.	Hospital costs exclude both items.
12. *Medical research*: All medical-research costs are included. The costs of research undertaken by the pharmaceutical and medical-supply industries are included through the price of products.	✔	✔	✔	✔
13. *Transport*: Ambulance costs are included, as are the transport costs of the health-care agencies. Personal travel costs incurred by patients are excluded.	✔	✔	Personal travel costs are included if (as is commonly the case) they are recognized by social security for reimbursement.	As for France.
14. *Capital construction*: Capital construction costs are included by two main methods: (1) directly, when incurred; or (2) via amortization charges. The variations are noted. In all cases private-sector capital costs are mainly recovered via charges for services.	Direct method.	Mainly direct, but some amortization of equipment. No double counting.	Mixture of the two methods. No double counting. Some public-sector capital construction costs are excluded.	Direct method.

Italy	Netherlands	Sweden	Switzerland	United Kingdom	United States
✓	✓	✓	✓	✓	✓
✓	✓	✓	✓	✓	✓
✓	These costs are excluded.	✓	✓	✓	✓
✓	✓	✓	✓	✓	✓
Hospital costs include both items.	Hospital costs exclude private fees. They include hospital-based ambulatory care.	Hospital costs include both items.	Hospital costs include both items, but hospitals undertake relatively little ambulatory care.	Hospital costs include both items.	Hospital costs exclude private fees. They include hospital-based ambulatory care.
Some medical-research costs may be excluded when the research is undertaken outside hospitals.	Medical-research costs are largely excluded.	✓	✓	✓	✓
✓	Costs of taxis are included when authorized by a physician.	✓	Even ambulance costs are probably largely excluded.	✓	✓
Mainly via amortization based on historic costs, plus interest at the actual rate incurred.	Mainly via amortization based on historic costs.	Direct method (amortization is also separately calculated for national-accounts purposes).	Similar to Canada.	Direct method.	Mixture of the two methods. Some (relatively small) double counting.

Table 2-1 *(continued)*

General Position (Standard Definition)	Australia	Canada	France	West Germany
15. *Deficits*: There are no hidden deficits of consequence.	✔	✔	✔	✔
16. *Administration*: Administration costs are included for hospitals and other health-care agencies, for government departments of health, and for health-insurance organizations. For social security and similar agencies, concerned with other functions besides health insurance, administrative costs are apportioned between functions. Costs of government departments other than health (for example, ministries of works and of finance) are excluded.	✔	✔	✔	Ministry costs are excluded.
17. *Value-added tax and similar taxes*: Value-added tax is charged in some countries and not in others, as noted.	No value-added tax. Small elements of payroll tax and sales tax on supplies used in private sector. Overall impact estimated at less than 0.5 percent of total health-care expenditure.	No value-added tax. Most goods and materials subject to 12 percent tax at manufacturers' level. Retail sales tax at 5 percent in most provinces; but virtually all health-care items are exempt, except drugs purchased without prescription.	Value-added tax levied only on retail sales of drugs, spectacles, appliances, and similar items. The rate prior to July 1976 was 20 percent. Overall impact perhaps 2 percent.	Value-added tax at 12 percent on certain items, including drugs purchased without prescription. Physicians' fees, prescribed drugs, and charges for public hospitals and nursing homes are all zero-rated. A reduced rate applies to some other items (such as appliances). Overall impact up to 3 percent.
Comment on overall comparability	Possibly slightly low (see 3 and 17).	Comparable.	Comparable.	Comparable (but note the spa problem and the possibly above-average impact of value-added tax).

Italy	Netherlands	Sweden	Switzerland	United Kingdom	United States
Figures have been adjusted to try to eliminate deficits and "artificial" interest charges.	✔	✔	✔	✔	✔
Administrative costs in provinces and communes are excluded.	✔	Costs of administering the health insurance plan are excluded (but the plan contributes less than 15 percent of total health-care finance).	Government costs are excluded, and the costs of administering health insurance are partly excluded.	✔	✔
In 1974 and 1975 all medical goods and services were subject to value-added tax, at 6 percent on drugs and 12 percent on physicians' fees and hospital services. Overall impact up to 10 percent.(?)	Value-added tax is not levied on the fees of physicians, dentists, and so on, nor on hospital care or patients' transport. It is levied at 4 percent on drugs, artificial limbs, hospital food, and some other items, and at 18 percent on buildings and equipment. Overall, estimated to account for 2.5 to 3 percent of total expenditure.	Value-added tax is levied on purchases of goods and services, including purchases by government. Sales taxes are levied on drugs purchased without prescription. Value-added tax and sales taxes amount to about 2 percent of total health-care expenditures.	The amount of value-added tax included is negligible since the major items of expenditure are all zero-rated.	Value-added tax is levied on a range of supplies, equipment and services, except for drugs supplied by a pharmacist against a prescription. I estimate that value-added tax accounted for 1½ to 2 percent of total 1975 expenditure.	No value-added tax but a varying State sales tax averaging about 5 percent. Not levied on physicians' fees nor on public sector. Overall impact less than 2 percent.
Probably low (see 3, 12, and 16, and note the fragmented nature of the data system; on the other hand, note 17).	Low by up to 5 percent (see 9).	Comparable	Certainly low. (See 3, 13, and 17. Also, data sources are fragmented, and there are substantial direct payments by consumers, which are difficult to capture in recorded costs.)	Comparable.	Comparable.

3 Health-Care Expenditures in Total

In the ten countries studied, total health-care spending from all sources, public and private, ranged in 1975 from a high of $717 (U.S. dollars) in Sweden to a low of $224 in Italy (see figure 3-1 and table 3-1). Behind this simple statement lie two difficulties: (1) What rates of exchange should be used in converting currencies? and (2) Are the definitions of total spending comparable between countries?

The exchange rates used are shown in the notes to table 3-1. They represent the average rate prevailing between the dollar and each of the other currencies in calendar 1975. For interest, table 3-2 shows comparisons based on the rates prevailing on 31 December 1975 and on 1 January 1979. (The 1 January 1979 conversion is not a defensible method of equating 1975 costs but was used to test the effect of the marked changes in exchange rates against the dollar that have taken place in recent years.) Using 1975 end-year rates makes relatively little difference to national-health expenditures stated in dollars, but the 1 January 1979 rates dramatically alter the expenditures of strong-currency countries, particularly Switzerland, West Germany, and the Netherlands. The average rate prevailing in the period (figure 3-1 and table 3-1) seems the fairest method of comparison, but one must bear in mind its limitations. Sharp fluctuations can occur and, as every traveler knows, money goes further in some places (such as the United Kingdom, Italy, and, more recently, the United States) than in others (Germany and Switzerland) at the official exchange rates, reflecting relative skepticism about the stability of the currency concerned. Within countries there are also substantial variations in relative prices, for example in the ratio of physicians' earnings to average earnings, as will be shown in table 4-7. But this is not the point emphasized here, which is simply that the general level of prices can be quite different in one country than in another when translated at the official rate of exchange. These limitations strengthen the argument for using other yardsticks, such as proportions of the gross national product (GNP), and for not placing too much weight on dollar comparisons.

The question of what constitutes health-care spending in different countries is even more difficult and haunts anyone who has worked in this field. Are the costs of training doctors, nurses, and others classified as health costs or as education? Where does the frontier lie between health spending and welfare, particularly in residential provision for the elderly and in services

Table 3-1
Total Health-Care Expenditures, Public and Private, Capital and Current, Calendar-Year 1975

	Australia[a]	Canada	France	West Germany	Italy	Netherlands	Sweden	Switzerland	United Kingdom[a]	United States
U.S. dollars per head	464	508	518	638	224	491	717	599	226	607
Current	432	482	NA[b]	609	NA	455	667	557	210	584
Capital	32	26	NA	29	NA	36	50	42	16	23
Percentage of GNP	7.3	7.1	7.9	9.4	7.1	8.1	8.5	6.9	5.5	8.6
Current	6.8	6.7	NA	9.0	NA	7.5	7.9	6.4	5.1	8.3
Capital	0.5	0.4	NA	0.4	NA	0.6	0.6	0.5	0.4	0.3
Percentage of GDP	7.3	7.0	8.2	9.4	7.1	8.1	8.5	7.1	5.5	8.7
Current	6.8	6.6	NA	9.0	NA	7.5	7.9	6.6	5.1	8.4
Capital	0.5	0.4	NA	0.4	NA	0.6	0.6	0.5	0.4	0.3

Notes:

1. *Exchange rates*: The exchange rates used in converting foreign currencies into U.S. dollars are averages for calendar 1975, derived from International Monetary Fund (IMF) Datastream. The rates are:

Units of Local Currency to U.S. $1

Australia	0.7632
Canada	1.0172
France	4.2864
Germany	2.4605
Italy	652.85
Netherlands	2.5292
Sweden	4.1522
Switzerland	2.5813
United Kingdom	0.4500

2. *Total health-care expenditure per capita:* The figures for each country are derived from the national summaries. In six cases no adjustment is necessary. Thus:

	1975 Figure from National Summary	1975 Figure in U.S. Dollars
Canada (Canadian dollars)	517	508
France (francs)	2,222	518
Germany (Deutschmarks)	1,571	638
Italy (lire)	146,265	224
Sweden (kronor)	2,978	717
Switzerland (Swiss francs)	1,546	599

The U.S. national summary is for fiscal years to 30 September. But DHEW supplied calendar-year figures, prepared on the same definitions, of $606.94 for 1975 and $681.35 for 1976. The Australian summary is also for fiscal years, in this case to 30 June. The 1974-1975 figure is Australian $314 and the 1975-1976 figure is Australian $395. Taking calendar 1975 as the average of the two fiscal years gives Australian $354.5 or U.S. $464. For the Netherlands the national summary is based on 1974 figures. Expenditure for 1975 is given as 16,992 million guilders in table 1.1 of the ministry's *Health Care in the Netherlands: Financial Analysis 1973-83*, which derives from the same sources as my 1974 figures. The 1975 total is equivalent to 1,243 florins per head or U.S. $491. Finally, the figures for the United Kingdom are for fiscal years ending 31 March: £83 for 1974-1975 and £107.9 for 1975-1976. If calendar 1975 is taken as a combination of these two in the ratio 25:75, then it equals approximately £102 per capita or U.S. $226.

3. *The breakdown between current and capital expenditure:* This is derived by using the percentages in table 4-3. The "buildings" percentage in that table (line 3) was used to estimate capital expenditure in dollars. Thus for Australia 7 percent of total health-care expenditure was on buildings: 7 percent of $464 is approximately $32. Current expenditure was obtained by deduction. No breakdown is available from table 4-3 for France and Italy.

4. *Total health-care expenditure as a percentage of GNP and of GDP:* As with expenditure per head, these figures are basically derived from the national summaries. The following are extracted directly from the tables without requiring adjustment:

	Percentage of GNP	Percentage of GDP
Canada	7.1	7.0
France	(7.9)*	8.2
West Germany	9.4	9.4
Italy	7.1	7.1
Sweden	8.5	8.5
Switzerland	6.9	7.1

*Estimated from GDP, using the 1974 relationship between GNP and GDP.

Table 3-1 *(continued)*

For Australia the GDP percentages are calculated in the national summary for the fiscal years (to 30 June) 1974-1975 and 1975-1976. They are, respectively, 7.0 and 7.6, implying a calendar 1975 figure of 7.3. GNP is not available for Australia but is thought to be not significantly different from GDP. Accordingly, 7.3 has also been taken as the GNP average.

The Netherlands' GNP and GDP percentages for 1974 are given in the national summary. The 1975 percentages were derived from more recent ministry statistics in the same series (see note 2).

As mentioned in note 2, U.K. health-care expenditure for calendar 1975 is estimated at approximately £102 per capita, from the fiscal-year figures of £83 in fiscal 1974-1975 and £107.9 in 1975-1976. GNP and GDP are known for calendar 1975 as £1,855 and £1,841 per capita respectively. £102 represents 5.50 percent of GNP and 5.54 percent of GDP, or (rounding to one decimal place) 5.5 percent in both cases.

For the United States, DHEW supplied calendar-year figures of 8.6 percent of GNP for 1975 and 8.8 percent for 1976. The percentage of GDP for 1975 was estimated using IMF statistics for the relationship between U.S. GDP and U.S. GNP that year.

[a]Estimated from figures for fiscal 1975 and fiscal 1976.

[b]NA means that the breakdown between capital and current is not available.

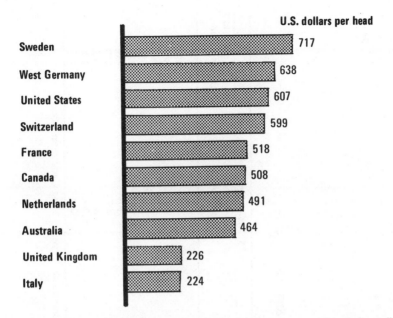

U.S. dollars per head

Sweden	717
West Germany	638
United States	607
Switzerland	599
France	518
Canada	508
Netherlands	491
Australia	464
United Kingdom	226
Italy	224

Source: Table 3-1, which gives an estimated breakdown between current and capital spending.

Figure 3-1. Total Health-Care Expenditures (Public and Private, Capital and Current) in 1975

for the elderly and handicapped? Which of the reported costs include value-added tax, and does this distort the comparisons? These questions of definition are discussed in chapter 2 (see particularly table 2-1). In brief, there are important differences between countries, mainly affecting specific cost categories within the totals rather than total health-care expenditures. Because of differences in definition, the total for Switzerland is (in my opinion) 5 to 10 percent low, and those for Australia, Italy, and the Netherlands up to 5 percent low. The one major area of uncertainty concerns the boundary with social welfare in the care of the elderly and handicapped, where the boundary is by its nature blurred and the classification used in national accounts somewhat arbitrary. The impact on recorded health-care expenditures could be substantial.

Using basically the same sources, classifications and methods, the estimates of total health-care expenditures in U.S. dollars have been recalculated for 1977. The results are shown in figure 3-2.

Relationships and Trends

As previous studies have documented [6, 8, 27] there is a clear relationship between health-care spending and national income. For 1975 this is il-

Table 3-2
Impact of Varying Exchange Rates on Health-Care Expenditures Stated in U.S. Dollars

Country	1975 Expenditure (Local Currency)	U.S. Dollar Equivalents		
		At 1975 Average Exchange Rate	At 31 December 1975 Exchange Rate	At 1 January 1979 Exchange Rate
Sweden	2,978 kronor	717	679	696
West Germany	1,571 Deutschmarks	638	599	863
United States	607 U.S. dollars	607	607	607
Switzerland	1,546 Swiss francs	599	590	955
France	2,222 francs	518	495	533
Canada	517 Canadian dollars	508	509	437
Netherlands	1,243 guilders	491	462	630
Australia	354 Australian dollars	464	445	407
United Kingdom	102 pounds	226	206	208
Italy	146,265 lire	224	214	177

Sources: Table 3-1 and National Data Summaries. Exchange rates are from the International Monetary Fund Datastream service.

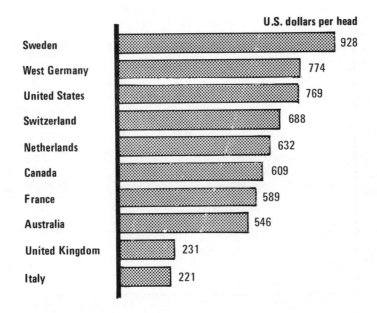

U.S. dollars per head

Sweden	928
West Germany	774
United States	769
Switzerland	688
Netherlands	632
Canada	609
France	589
Australia	546
United Kingdom	231
Italy	221

Source: Updated estimates calculated on the same basis as those in table 3-1, converted to U.S. dollars at the average exchange rate prevailing in calendar 1977.

Figure 3-2. Total Health-Care Expenditures (Public and Private, Capital and Current) in 1977

lustrated by figure 3-3. The higher a country's GNP, the higher tends to be its health-care spending, expressed in U.S. dollars per capita. This is not surprising, although it immediately suggests something fundamental about health-care expenditure. There is no constant and inevitable level of health-services provision. On the contrary, the amount spent in each country is very strongly influenced by the means available.

The correlation between per-capita health-care spending and GNP (at market prices) in figure 3-3 is well over 0.9—a finding confirmed by others [27]. The fit is marginally improved (from 0.919 to 0.938) if health-care expenditures for Switzerland, Italy, the Netherlands, and Australia are adjusted as suggested from table 2-1 (by 7.5 percent in the case of Switzerland, and 2.5 percent for each of the other three countries). Put another way, knowing a country's GNP per capita and nothing else, one can predict its health-care expenditure within close limits. Although from this study one can only make this statement about the Western developed countries included in it, from Abel-Smith [6] it appears to apply to some degree also to developing countries and to the communist bloc. Within any of these groups, however, there are countries that do not fit so neatly into the pattern.

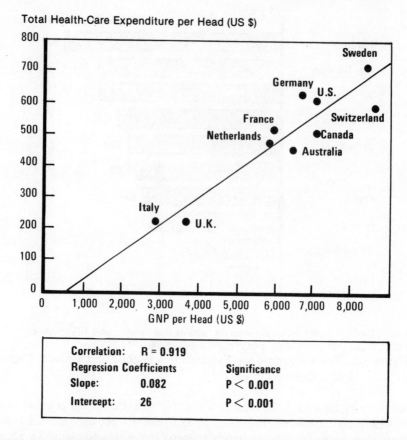

Source: Table 3-1 for health-care expenditures. *World Bank Atlas*, 1978 for GNP per capita for 1975. In all cases GNP is at market prices.

Note: There are some discrepancies between the *World Bank Atlas* figures for GNP, used on the horizontal axis, and GNP figures extracted from the national data summaries and converted to U.S. dollars at the average rate of exchange. In four cases the resulting figures vary less than 1 percent and in another three by 2.5 percent or less. For France, Italy, and the United Kingdom, on the other hand, the national summary figure for GNP at market prices is 6 to 9 percent *higher* than the World Bank estimate. I cannot explain this. Possibly the World Bank figures for these countries will be increased in later editions of the *Atlas*, since upward adjustment has been quite common previously.

Figure 3-3. Total Health-Care Expenditures and GNP, 1975

If health-care expenditures from all sources are expressed as a proportion of GNP, as in figures 3-4 and 3-5, instead of in dollars per capita, the variation among countries is substantially less. The figures can be compared with those in the Organization for Economic Cooperation and Development (OECD) study [8] and, for five countries, with those of Abel-Smith

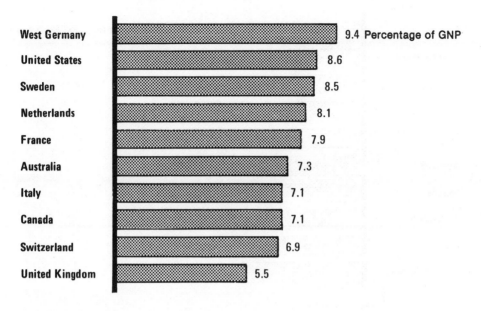

Source: Table 3-1.

Figure 3-4. Total Health-Care Expenditures (Public and Private) as a Proportion of GNP in 1975

and Maynard [9]. (In the OECD study, see tables 1 and 10 on pages 10 and 26, and in Abel-Smith and Maynard, table 1 on page B-4.) Precise comparisons are difficult because of variations in years and in definitions. Generally, my figures are higher than those in either of the other two studies, particularly for West Germany, Italy, and (in the OECD case) Switzerland. Only for the Netherlands is my figure somewhat lower, perhaps reinforcing the suggestion made in table 2-1 and in the text that my estimate is low in this instance. Abel-Smith and Maynard essentially relied on existing official estimates, which were in many cases incomplete. The OECD study focused mainly on *public* expenditure, and its estimates of total spending may also be somewhat low. There is no disagreement among us about broad trends.

There is a tendency (illustrated in figures 3-6 and 3-7) for the wealthier countries to spend more on health care, not merely in dollar terms but, more interestingly, as a proportion of GNP. Figure 3-7 illustrates that for nine of the countries, excluding Switzerland (where the information is weak), the relationship holds also for 1965 and 1970. Moreover, as Brian Abel-Smith also observed [6], for at least the last twenty years every country has tended to increase the proportion of its GNP devoted to health care.

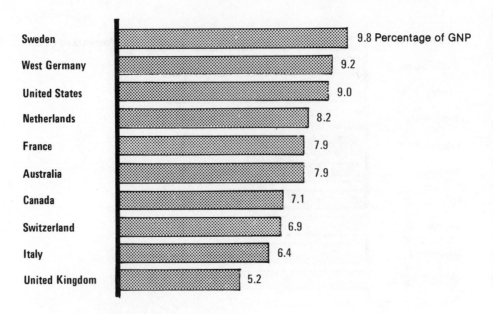

Source: Table 3-3.

Figure 3-5. Total Health-Care Expenditures (Public and Private) as a Proportion of GNP in 1977

Figures comparable with those collected in this study for 1975 are not
uniformly available for the whole period for every country surveyed, but
nevertheless the evidence for the broad trend is incontrovertible (see figures
3-8, 3-9, and 3-10 and table 3-3). This historical trend may be the result of
rising prosperity; in other words, the relationship shown across countries in
figures 3-6 and 3-7 may also apply in the same country through time as GNP
rises. The evidence from the United States (figure 3-10) supports this
hypothesis, with a very high correlation between GNP per capita and the
percentage of GNP spent on health care in recent years. However, Canada
in the 1970s provides an interesting exception (to which we will return) to
the broad trend in figures 3-8 and 3-9.

Causes of Increased Spending

The sharp, continuing rise in health-care spending has attracted attention
around the world; and volumes have already been written about it [21, 24].
Although every author has a unique way of describing the causes, there is a
substantial measure of agreement about them. Six main causes can be identified:

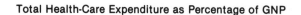

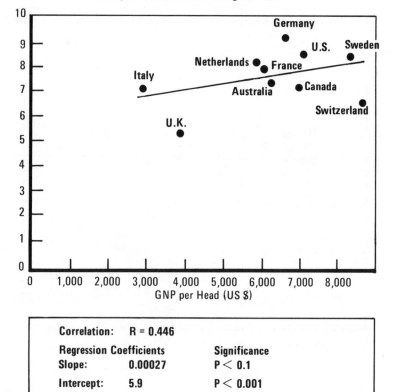

Source: Table 3-1 for health-care expenditures as a percentage of GNP. *World Bank Atlas*, 1978 for per-capita GNP.

Figure 3-6. Total Health-Care Expenditures as a Proportion of GNP by GNP, 1975

1. *Demographic changes* producing populations that are older on average, live mainly in cities, and do less manual work. Average age has risen, through falling birth rates and reduced child mortality. Beyond childhood, life expectancy has altered comparatively little, but many more people are surviving into old age. These demographic changes have contributed to the changing pattern of disease and have, in general, increased expenditure since (as we shall see) costs of health care are high for the older age groups.

2. *A changing pattern of disease* toward chronic illness and handicap associated with aging, speeded or slowed by personal behavior, and an increased awareness and concern about psychiatric illness. Such health prob-

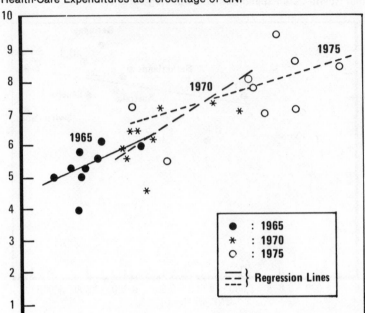

Source: Table 3-3 for health-care expenditures as a percentage of GNP. *World Bank Atlas*, 1967, 1972, and 1977 for per-capita GNP.

Figure 3-7. Health-Care Expenditures as Percentage of GNP Plotted against GNP per Capita for Nine Countries and Three Years

lems as these are not quickly resolved by medical intervention. Perhaps we have become overreliant on medical care for alleviation and comfort. However, if we are dependent on continuing medical intervention, we should not be too surprised at cumulative expense.

3. *Advances in medical technology* and the introduction of far more sophisticated patterns of diagnosis and care, particularly in the acute-hospital sector. Such advances are frequently expensive, at least initially, as medicine reaches out to tackle ever more complex problems. Only in rare instances, such as the conquest of tuberculosis and the prevention of polio, do they result in substantial net savings. Much more often the effect is to extend the scope of medical care and to increase costs.

4. *Rising public and professional expectations* connected with technological advance and also concerning the less-scientific aspects of care.

Table 3-3
Trends in Total Health-Care Expenditures (percentage of GNP)

Year	Australia[a]	Canada	France	West Germany	Italy	Netherlands	Sweden	Switzerland	United Kingdom	United States
1950		4.0	(3.4)				3.4		3.9	4.4
1955		4.3	(4.5)			(4.0)	4.1		3.4	4.4
1960	(5.0)	5.6	(4.7)			(4.5)	4.7		3.8	5.3
1965	(5.2)	6.1	(5.8)		(5.0)	(5.3)	5.6	(3.8)	3.9	6.1
1970	5.5	7.1	6.4	6.4		6.3	7.4		4.3	7.6
1971		7.4	6.6	7.0	(6.1)		7.9		4.3	7.8
1972	6.1	7.2	6.7	7.3		7.2	8.0		4.5	8.0
1973	6.0	6.8	6.8	7.8		7.5	7.8		4.4	7.9
1974	6.0	6.7	(7.1)	8.6	6.7	7.7	8.1	(5.7)	5.1	8.2
1975	7.0	7.1	7.9	9.4	7.1	8.1	8.5		5.5	8.6
1976	7.6	7.1	7.9	9.3		8.1	8.8	6.9	5.4	8.7
1977	(7.7)	7.1	7.9	9.2	6.4	8.2	9.8		5.2	8.9
1978	8.0		8.2	9.2				6.9	5.2	8.9
1979			8.4						5.2	9.0

Sources: The sources of these time series are basically the same as those used in the national summaries, and are therefore comparable with the 1975 figures in table 3-1. However, I have not researched them in the same detail as I have the national summaries. They should be reliable as an indicator of changes over time in the country concerned, but not necessarily for comparison across countries in a particular year.

Note: figures in parentheses are approximations not derived from primary sources

1. *Australia:* The source is J.S. Deeble, *Health Expenditure in Australia 1960-61 to 1975-76* (Canberra: ANC, 1978), and the series is for fiscal years to 30 June. His table 4, p. 25, gives total health-care expenditures as a percentage of GDP. GNP is not available for Australia, but it is thought that it would not differ materially from GDP. My 1960 and 1965 percentages are estimated from this series, which does not have a figure for either year. For 1974-1975 and 1975-1976, see the national summary. 1976-1977 and 1977-1978 are from *Australia Health Expenditure 1974-75-1977-78: An Analysis* (Canberra: Australian government, June 1980).

2. *Canada:* All figures were supplied by Health, and Welfare Canada, Health Economics and Data Analysis Division. 1977 figures are rough estimates only.

3. *France:* The definition of health-care expenditures used in the present study corresponds with ''La dépense nationale de santé au sens large'' as defined by CREDOC in its studies up to and including 1975. The 1975 figure of 117,215 million francs, as used in table 3-1 and the national summary, is documented in detail in CREDOC's publication of December 1977, entitled *La Dépense Nationale de Santé en 1975*. For 1975 GNP is not available for France: the percentage was therefore estimated assuming the 1974 relationship between GDP and GNP (GDP = 96.4/100 × GNP).

Table 3-3 (continued)

The GNP percentages for 1970 to 1973, inclusive, are given in CREDOC's *La Dépense Nationale de Santé 1971-1972-1973*, p. 75. In these years the relationship between *consommation médicale finale* (which covers medical care only and excludes education, research, preventive activities, and administration) and *dépense nationale de santé au sens large* was stable at approximately 85 percent. I have used this ratio to estimate figures for 1950, 1955, 1960, and 1965, using CREDOC's records of *consommation médicale finale* as a percentage of GNP for those years. For 1974 the calculation was similar. Recently, CREDOC has changed its definitions in two main ways, following an extensive review of its methodology published in 1979 under the title *Comptes Nationaux de la Santé*. CREDOC now excludes from hospitalization costs charges for residential care of handicapped children (3,177 million francs in 1975). It also excludes the costs of social-security administration attributed to health care (9,556 million francs in 1975). Both these items are typical examples of definitional problems at the boundary of health-care expenditures (see chapter 2 of this book). CREDOC's estimates for *dépense nationale de santé* in 1975, 1976, and 1977 have been adjusted to include these items so that they are comparable with earlier figures used in the present study. For 1978 and 1979 my estimates are based on CREDOC's provisional figures for *consommation médicale finale* (CMF). The ratio of CMF to *dépense nationale de santé* in the new, narrower definition is likely to have remained stable at about 93:100, which was the approximate ratio in 1970 and 1976. I have used this ratio and have also estimated the upward adjustments for the two changes in definitions discussed above. For all years later than 1974 I have assumed that GNP, if published, would have maintained a stable relationship with GDP on the basis that GDP = 96.4/100 × GNP.

4. *West Germany*: 1974 and 1975 figures are supported in the national summary. They were obtained from Statistisches Bundesamt, Wiesbaden, by excluding cash benefits from the statistics in *Die Struktur der Ausgaben im Gesundheitsbereich und ihre Entwicklung seit 1970*. Figures for 1970-1973 inclusive and for 1976-1978 were also supplied by Statistisches Bundesamt on a comparable basis.

5. *Italy*: The source for the Italian figures is the Istituto per la ricerca di Economia Sanitaria in Milan. 1974 and 1975 figures are detailed in the national summary. Figures for 1965 and 1970 are rough estimates, intended to be comparable, supplied by the institute. The reduction in GNP terms between 1975 and 1977 follows several moves by government to limit the increase in health-care expenditures. It is, however, possible that there has been an unrecorded increase in private expenditures during this period, to circumvent government controls. If so, the 1977 figure may prove to be an underestimate.

6. *Netherlands*: For the 1974 percentage, see the national summary. The 1974 figures were supplied by the Ministerie van Volksgezondheid en Milieuhygiene at Leidschendam. As explained in the notes, they exclude self-medication (nonprescribed drugs), which are included for all other countries. Figures for 1970, 1972, and 1973 come from the same source and are comparable. For 1955, 1960, and 1965 the figures are rough indicators only, derived by me from the previous Netherlands series which excluded expenditure on institutions for the mentally handicapped and on nursing homes. The percentages of GNP excluding these two items were:

	Percentage of GNP
1953	3.3
1958	3.9
1963	4.3
1968	5.3
1970	5.6

For 1970 the relationship between the two definitions was 6.3/5.6 = 1.125. To make some allowance for the rapid increase in nursing home beds in the late 1960s, I have reduced the ratio to 1.1 for the earlier years, and applied that to estimate the missing figures. For 1975 to 1977 the figures are on the same basis of definitions as for 1974. The expenditure totals lying behind them are documented in table 1.1 of *Health Care in the Netherlands: Financial Analysis, 1973-83*, published by the ministry in September 1979. In that publication the 1974 figure is somewhat lower (7.5 percent) than the 7.7 percent used by me, owing to statistical corrections since my study was carried out.

7. *Sweden*: The complete series was supplied by the National Central Bureau of Statistics in Stockholm to comply with the definitions used in this study. The series was calculated in terms of GDP, because of lack of consistent information for GNP. However, analysis for 1974 and 1975 (see the national summary) shows that the difference between GDP and GNP was extremely small for Sweden in those two years.

8. *Switzerland*: Swiss figures are particularly hard to obtain. As explained in the national summary, I am indebted to Pierre Gygi for the 1975 figures, which are documented in Pierre Gygi and Heiner Henny, *Le système suisse de santé: dépenses, structure et formation des prix dans le domaine des soins médicaux* (Bern: Hans Huber, 1977). The figures exclude ambulance costs, which are included for all other countries. The 1965 and 1973 percentages given in table 3-3 are rough indicators only. They are based on earlier, detailed studies by Gygi for those two years, with very approximate adjustment to allow for figures that are now known to have been omitted from them. The 1977 figures are based on Gygi and Henny, *Das schweizerische Gesundheitswesen* (Bern: Hans Huber, 1980).

9. *United Kingdom*: The U.K. expenditures for fiscal 1974-1975 and 1975-1976 are calculated in detail in the national summary. I have adjusted them approximately to a calendar-year basis, as explained in the notes to table 3-1, by taking an approximate fraction of each fiscal year's expenditure, and relating the resulting health-care expenditure per capita to GNP per capita for the calendar year. My estimates include (besides National Health Service expenditure) spending on medical care for the armed forces, medical research funded outside the NHS, the costs of private medical care incurred by U.K. residents, and spending on nonprescribed drugs. Expenditures for 1950-1974 inclusive have been estimated from government figures for NHS expenditures and direct payments by patients, Lee Donaldson's figures for private insurance [for example Lee Donaldson Associates *UK Private Medical Care: Provident Schemes Statistics 1978* (London: July 1979)], and Office of Health Economics figures for OTC drugs. These figures account for 97-97.5 percent of totals in the years for which my estimates are complete. I have assumed the same relationship in earlier years. 1977 and 1978 are estimated from *National Income and Expenditure*, 1979 edition, for NHS expenditures and updated figures for each of the other elements included in my estimates for 1975 and 1976. 1979 is similarly estimated from *National Income and Expenditure*, 1980 edition.

10. *United States*: The U.S. series is from R.M. Gibson, "National Health Expenditures, Fiscal Year 1979" *Health Care Financing Review* (Summer 1980): table 1.

[a]Fiscal years end 30 June.

Percentage of GNP

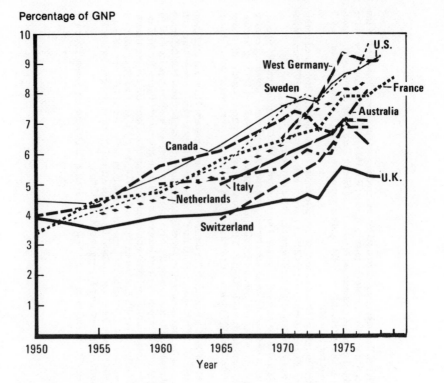

Source: Table 3-3.

Figure 3-8. Trends in Total Health-Care Spending as a Proportion of GNP

Ideas change about what constitute appropriate and acceptable living standards, not merely in general hospitals but for groups like the mentally ill, the handicapped, and the elderly, who have often been neglected in the past. (To say that expectations have risen does not deny that some standards of care may actually have fallen, for example through loss of continuity.) Among the changes in expectations has been an increased reliance on formal health services, rather than on informal coping mechanisms in the family and the community. Tasks have been transferred to the formal health-care providers.

5. *Higher wage and salary costs* caused in part by a catching-up process of health-sector wages, including the trend toward equal pay for women. Another factor is increased specialization and higher skill levels, connected with technological change and with the aspirations of staff. Higher costs are also the inevitable result of failures to achieve manpower savings in the health sector in a world in which manpower is becoming ever more expensive. In health care, although technological advances may well have helped

	Australia[a]	Canada	France	West Germany	Italy	Netherlands	Sweden	Switzerland	United Kingdom	United States
1950		4.0	(3.4)				3.4		3.9	4.5
1955		4.3	(4.5)			(4.0)	4.1		3.4	4.4
1960	(5.0)	5.6	(4.7)			(4.5)	4.7		3.8	5.3
1965	(5.2)	6.1	(5.8)		(5.0)	(5.3)	5.6	(3.8)	3.9	6.2
1970	5.5	7.1	6.4	6.4	(6.1)[b]	6.3	7.4		4.3	7.6
1975	7.0	7.1	7.9	9.4	7.1	8.1	8.5	6.9	5.5	8.6
1977	(7.9)	7.1	7.9	9.2	6.4	8.2	9.8	6.9	5.2	8.9
1978	8.0		8.2	9.2					5.2	8.9
1979			8.4						5.2	9.0

Source: Table 3-3.

Note: Figures in brackets are approximate, not derived from primary sources.

[a]Fiscal years to 30 June for Australia.

[b]1971.

Figure 3-9. Trends in Total Health-Care Spending as a Percentage of GNP

people who could not be helped previously, they have seldom resulted in manpower reductions; whereas in other sectors technological investment has increased the quantity of output per person and hence has permitted pay rates to be increased and working hours reduced. These higher manpower costs in other sectors sooner or later affect pay in the health sector.

6. *A transfer of financing* from direct payment by individuals to insurance schemes and to government. An intended effect of this transfer has been to remove the barrier to access for those who could not afford to pay, and to a substantial extent this result has been achieved. In the process, naturally enough, a boost has been given to the supply side of health services. Particularly when public insurance is used, no one is in a position to control such an expansion. It must be said, however, that in countries like France, the United States, and Switzerland there is still substantial variation in the use of services by different income groups, suggesting that there still are income-related barriers to access. Even in the United Kingdom, after thirty years of a National Health Service virtually free at the time of use, the evidence suggests that poorer people make less use of health services *relative to their needs* than do the more prosperous [30].

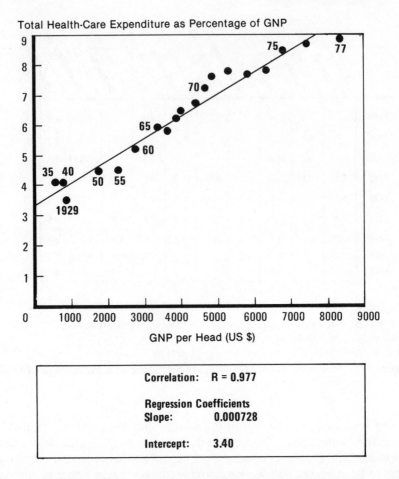

Source: *Department of Health, Education, and Welfare, Social Security Bulletin* (Washington, D.C.: July 1978) table 1.
Figure 3-10. Health-Care Expenditures as Percentage of GNP, Plotted Against GNP per Capita (United States, 1929-1977)

Most of these causes will continue to operate in the future. It is true that in some countries, including the United Kingdom, the movement to public funding has gone almost as far as it can go. But the swing to more chronic disease and handicap is by no means finished; indeed, the more successful medicine is with one set of problems, the more intractable the next set is likely to be. And the demographic trends are still set toward rising cost, since the proportion of those over 75, with their high level of health-care needs, is still rising throughout the developed world; even a rapid increase in birth rate would not improve the situation, since the very young are another expensive group in health-care terms (see figure 3-11). Moreover, the pressures of medical technology and of rising expectations have certainly not spent their strength. Indeed, one cannot rely in the future on the size of savings from medical technology that have occurred in the case of tuberculosis, infectious diseases, and the inpatient treatment of psychiatric patients. Except for these savings, the rise in overall health-care expenditures would have been sharper than it was, especially in the 1950s. Moreover, the health sector remains, and is always likely to remain, labor intensive. Anyone who believes that health-care expenditures have increased in the past simply because no one was watching them, and that the stealthy advances will stop once they are spotted, is fooling himself.

The Response of Governments

However, there certainly is more resistance to further increases in health-care expenditures than existed a few years ago. It was clear that there would ultimately be such resistance [29]. The inevitable clash with other priorities has come sooner and more sharply in North America and in continental Europe than expected, partly because of the sluggishness in the world economy and the effects of high inflation on the costs of public programs. Thus governments are applying the brakes to their health-care budgets as firmly as they judge politically possible. Canada provides the most ineresting example to date of what is also likely to happen to government-controlled expenditures elsewhere (see figure 3-12 and table 3-3).

   After a federally backed system of national insurance for physicians' fees was introduced in 1966, complementing a similar scheme for hospital insurance in 1958, there was a sharp increase in Canadian health-care spending until 1971. Federal and provincial governments were alarmed by the increase, in view of the large share of their budgets already devoted to health care (already more than 20 percent of government spending in some provinces) and the worsening economic background. They therefore sought to hold further increases to a minimum and have had some success in doing so, as figure 3-12 shows. Whether they can do so more than temporarily is more questionable. In any case, learning to control public health-care expenditures is not enough in itself. Control might be achieved at the expense of equity, or access, or quality of care, or all three.

Health and Public Policy

Health is not a field in which the invisible hand of the free market can safely be left to solve the problem of allocating scarce resources, with minimal

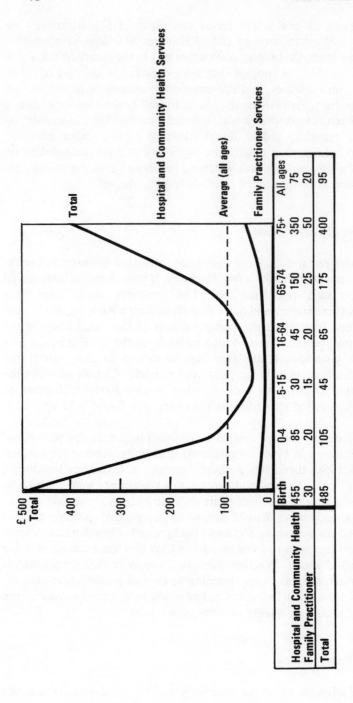

	Birth	0-4	5-15	16-64	65-74	75+	All ages
Hospital and Community Health	455	85	30	45	150	350	75
Family Practitioner	30	20	15	20	25	50	20
Total	485	105	45	65	175	400	95

Based on data from Command 7049 11 (London: HMSO, 1978), p. 85.

Note: Birth = cost per delivery, including pre- and postnatal care; this is exluded from the costs by age group.

Figure 3-11. Estimated Current Health-Care Expenditures by Age Group, in Pounds per Capita (United Kingdom 1975-1976)

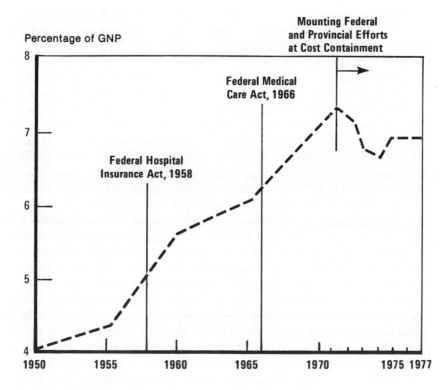

Source: Table 3-3.

Figure 3-12. Trend in Total Health-Care Spending in Canada

government intervention. There are three major snags in the application of demand and supply to health care. The first is that some of the principal decisions about utilization are not made by consumers but by providers. Once we have asked a doctor for help, it is chiefly doctors who decide what services we require; they are therefore among the prime determinants of how resources are used in the whole health sector. The United States supplies evidence that, for example, the incidence of surgery is strongly influenced by the availability, distribution, and motivation of surgeons [31]. In the health-care field, demand and supply are not independent forces reaching a point of equilibrium at which marginal benefits equal marginal costs, as in the classic market system. Instead, the quantity and quality of medical services tend to rise to the point where, in the judgment of providers, the marginal benefit of further services is zero. Put more simply, when doctors and hospitals are paid for each item of service, they no doubt ask themselves whether an additional item will benefit their patient, but they do not ask whether he (or the organization paying the bill on his behalf) would prefer to spend the money in some other way.

The second snag is that health care has become so expensive that only the very rich can afford to risk paying the full cost at the time of use. For the vast majority some form of insurance, or of public provision, is the only sensible course, so that the high cost for the few who need extensive medical care is borne by the many who draw lightly on their insurance. In such an arrangement, the link between decisions about utilization and the cost to the individual is tenuous. At the time of use individuals may be more inclined to seek value from their previous contributions than to minimize cost.

The third snag is that governments, reflecting our instincts as electors, are not prepared to see the interplay of market forces carried to a ruthless conclusion in health care. For what happens through the free interplay of market forces, in this as in other fields, is that the resources go where people can afford to pay for them and where suppliers find operation attractive. This can be seen clearly, for example, in the share of medical resources taken by northern Italy compared with the south, or by the Paris area compared with other parts of France [32]. Under a free-market system, those who cannot afford to pay, directly or through insurance, simply have less access to medical care. None of us is happy about this. We feel instinctively that in the health-care field the care given should be related to need rather than to the capacity to pay for it, or to its prestige or profitability to suppliers. And as soon as governments intervene to secure equity in health care for the less fortunate, they disturb the interaction of supply and demand. One cannot simultaneously remove the sting of deprivation and expect the free market to exercise constraint on the supply of medical care.

This does not mean that private enterprise has no role in the health-care field. Among outstanding examples of private-enterprise contributions are those of physicians (and other individual practitioners) in contract with a system, rather than employed by it; Health Maintenance Organizations (HMOs) and other forms of prepaid group practice for defined populations; and the research contribution of the pharmaceutical and medical-equipment industries. But it does mean that health indisputably becomes a major matter of public policy and of shared communal responsibility, involving patients, their families, those working in the health field, those responsible for sickness funds, and government. If the invisible hand does not work, or does not work acceptably, government should be concerned about far more complex matters than the size of the bills presented to it.

We have already seen that there have been very strong forces behind the increases in health-care expenditures, most of which have not spent their strength. The bills presented to health-insurance agencies and to government are a product of these forces. To check the increase in total health-care expenditure more than temporarily, government must understand and influence them. This provides one reason for looking, as we will in chapter 4, beyond total expenditure to how the money is spent in different countries.

Moreover, government cannot properly concern itself solely with expenditures without also considering value for money, which in the end means effectiveness. And assessing effectiveness in the health field poses some disconcerting difficulties. If effectiveness means impact on human suffering, handicap, and death, then impact can be made by prevention and by care as well as by cure, and may come from sources entirely outside the health-care field as traditionally defined [33]. The chief measurement difficulty arises from the heterogeneity of health needs and of the influences on them. At the level of a single disease or condition it may not be too difficult to assess the impact of a course of treatment (which is not to say that assessment at that level has received anything like the attention which it deserves [34]). But health needs are myriad and are very far from homogeneous, so that any overall assessment of effectiveness would have to take account of a very large number of such disease-specific measures. This raises problems not only of aggregation but also of weighting. If many measures are to be combined, their relative importance must first be determined.

Work is being done by health economists, social scientists, and epidemiologists on improved measures of need and impact [35]. Meanwhile, some limited hypotheses about value for money in national health-care expenditures can be formulated and are worth bearing in mind as we look in more detail at the makeup of health-care expenditures.

First, a high level of spending does not necessarily ensure high health status. If one takes a composite ranking of seventeen age- and sex-specific mortality rates (from perinatal mortality to death prior to age 65) for each of the ten countries, there is no consistent correlation between high levels of spending and low mortality rates in these groups. Although nations like Sweden and the Netherlands spend highly and enjoy excellent health status, West Germany and the United States spend equally highly and have a relatively low standard of health by these measures (see tables 3-4 and 3-5). This is not surprising in view of the other influences on health besides health services, and of the reasons why high spending may not represent high value. One could also legitimately argue that mortality rates are insensitive measures, particularly in relation to chronic disease and handicap. While this is perfectly true and is a good reason for pursuing better measures [35], it is unlikely to invalidate the broad hypothesis that high spending levels are not by themselves any guarantee of good results.

From a quite different perspective one can provide another illustration of this hypothesis. It has been characteristic of health-care systems in the developed countries in recent years that people employed in them expect

Table 3-4
Health-Care Expenditures and Health Status, Assessed by Seventeen
Age- and Sex-Specific Mortality Rates

Country	1975 Health-Care Expenditures as a Percentage of GNP		1975 Mortality Ranking A		1975 Mortality Ranking B	
	Percent	Rank	Standardized Index	Rank	Standardized Index	Rank
West Germany	9.4	1	1.23	10	1.23	10
United States	8.6	2	1.18	9	1.17	9
Sweden	8.5	3	0.76	1	0.73	1
Netherlands	8.1	4	0.80	2	0.79	2
France	7.9	5	1.11	8	1.10	7
Australia	7.3	6	1.01	5	1.02	5
Italy	7.1	7 =	1.04	6	1.11	8
Canada	7.1	7 =	1.08	7	1.06	6
Switzerland	6.9	9	0.86	3	0.84	3
United Kingdom	5.5	10	0.91	4	0.93	4

Source: Tables 3-1 and 3-5.
Note: Within each age- and sex-specific measure, the rate for each country has been divided by the mean for the ten countries. Thus (in the first line of table 3-5), the perinatal mortality rate for Sweden in 1975, at 11.1 per 1,000 live births, was 0.63 of the mean (17.60 per 1,000) for the ten countries in that year. Sweden's overall position in index A of table 3-4 represents the average of its positions, similarly calculated, on all seventeen measures. For index B the method is the same, except that infant and perinatal mortality are given three times the weight of other indicators on the grounds of their relatively greater importance.

shorter working hours (for example, reduced service loads for student nurses) or improved pay for traditional hours (as is the case with junior hospital doctors). Such changed expectations generate large increases in expenditure with little, if any, short-term benefit to patients.

Conversely, it would be unwise to assume that expenditure decisions are irrelevant to changes in health status. Returning to the Canadian example, when cost curbs were applied sharply by provincial governments in the early 1970s, hospital boards were exhorted to make savings without affecting standards of patient care. In the short term that can often be done by eliminating waste or extravagance and by postponing maintenance and similar items. There is undoubtedly also scope in the longer term for finding better, less-expensive solutions to some health-care problems, for example, through accident prevention and reductions in smoking and drinking. But tight financial constraints maintained over a long period could also slow down the pace of innovation, threaten standards, and open a widening gap between the level of service that is technically possible and that which is actually offered. Those who are cynical about the value of medical care may accept the reality of this danger while denying that it will have any harmful effect on health [36].   The effect is not easy to prove, and its investigation

**Table 3-5
Age- and Sex-Specific Mortality Rates (1975): Ratio of Each Country to the Mean Rate for Each Indicator**

	Mean Rate for the Ten Countries	Australia	Canada	France	West Germany	Italy	Netherlands	Sweden	Switzerland	United Kingdom	United States
Perinatal mortality (perinatal deaths per 1,000 live births)	17.60	1.09	0.94	1.11	1.10	1.37	0.80	0.63	0.77	1.02	1.18
Infant mortality (deaths in the first year per 1,000 live births)	14.45	0.99	1.04	1.02	1.36	1.45	0.73	0.57	0.74	0.98	1.11
Maternal mortality (maternal deaths per 100,000 live births)	15.01	0.37	0.63	1.47	2.64	2.09	0.34	0.13	0.63	0.85	0.85
Male 1-4	759.30	1.10	1.12	1.13	1.14	0.90	1.03	0.64	1.02	0.89	1.02
Female 1-4	592.30	1.11	1.11	1.07	1.20	1.00	1.00	0.66	0.90	0.88	1.07
Male 5-14	400.60	0.93	1.24	1.06	1.08	1.04	0.93	0.82	0.97	0.84	1.10
Female 5-14	264.80	0.93	1.19	1.04	1.10	0.96	0.93	0.96	1.06	0.80	1.03
Male 15-24	1,345.90	1.06	1.36	1.09	1.13	0.73	0.65	0.81	1.02	0.69	1.31
Female 15-24 (Deaths per annum per million in that age group)	484.50	1.03	1.22	1.16	1.19	0.81	0.70	0.81	0.98	0.82	1.25
Male 25-34	1,339.50	0.97	1.15	1.13	1.16	0.84	0.66	0.92	0.90	0.70	1.51
Female 25-34	651.80	1.02	1.08	1.12	1.15	0.89	0.81	0.95	0.84	0.88	1.31
Male 35-44	2,629.10	1.11	1.10	1.29	1.15	0.92	0.69	0.92	0.80	0.79	1.32
Female 35-44	1,482.20	1.08	1.04	1.04	1.08	0.89	0.85	0.88	0.82	1.01	1.28
Male 45-54	7,128.20	1.00	1.04	1.16	1.05	0.99	0.84	0.81	0.82	1.00	1.20
Female 45-54	3,758.20	1.07	1.04	0.98	1.11	0.92	0.85	0.87	0.78	1.14	1.21
Male 55-64	18,237.80	1.11	1.01	1.08	1.11	0.99	0.93	0.78	0.84	1.07	1.12
Female 55-64	8,728.50	1.11	1.04	0.92	1.12	0.99	0.85	0.84	0.81	1.16	1.16
Overall position—index A (equal weighting for all indicators)											
Total		17.25	18.38	18.89	20.87	17.75	13.59	13.00	14.69	15.53	20.04
Mean		1.01	1.08	1.11	1.23	1.04	0.80	0.76	0.86	0.91	1.18
Rank		5	7	8	10	6	2	1	3	4	9
Overall position—index B (infant and perinatal mortality weighted × 3)											
Weighted mean		1.02	1.06	1.10	1.23	1.11	0.79	0.73	0.84	0.93	1.17
Rank		5	6	7	10	8	2	1	3	4	9

Table 3-5 *(continued)*

Notes:

1. *Selection of indicators:* In default of reliable international data on morbidity and handicap, age- and sex-specific mortality rates provide the principal available comparisons of health status. I have taken seventeen such measures from perinatal mortality (which comprises deaths of the fetus after the twenty-eighth week of pregnancy and deaths during the first week of life) to deaths in the age group 55 to 64. It might be argued that "success" on one indicator would be bound to lead to low performance on others, but this is not the case, once death rates after age 64 are omitted. Thus Sweden has mortality rates below average for the ten countries for every single indicator. There is some, relatively minor, double counting between mortality rates, specifically between perinatal and infant mortality (which overlap for deaths in the first week of life) and between maternal mortality and female deaths in the childbearing age groups. It is certainly *not* assumed that national differences in health status, as measured by differences in these rates, necessarily or primarily stem from differences in health services. On the contrary, they are likely to be more strongly influenced by factors like life style, heredity, and the environment. What is assumed is that health-care activities should be related to, and seek to make impact on, health status.

2. *Sources of data:* The main source is WHO, specifically the *World Health Statistics Annual* for 1978, volume I, (Geneva: WHO, 1978) supplemented by the 1977 *Annual* for Canada, France, and Italy. There are some inconsistencies in the data, which represented the latest available when the analysis was done.

    a. Most rates are for 1975, but for Canada and France only 1974 figures were available. For Italy 1975 figures were available for perinatal and infant mortality, and 1974 figures for everything else.

    b. Rates quoted for the United Kingdom are in fact for England and Wales. These slightly flatter the United Kingdom, since rates for Scotland and Northern Ireland are less good. As England and Wales account for 88 percent of U.K. population, however, the difference is not large. Moreover, in the present context my point—that high expenditure does not guarantee high performance on these indicators—is not affected, since for England and Wales health-care expenditure per capita is appreciably lower relative to GNP than is health-care expenditure per capita in the rest of the United Kingdom.

    c. Maternal mortality rates are not given as such in the *World Health Statistics Annual.* They were computed from maternal-related deaths (International Classification of Diseases codes A112-A118) and live births.

3. *Method of calculation:* For each age- and sex-specific mortality rate the mean for the ten countries has been calculated. Then each country's rate has been divided by the mean. The result is a standardized index showing each country's position relative to the other nine. For example, for perinatal mortality the rates for the ten countries are:

	Perinatal Mortality per Thousand Live Births 1975
Australia	19.2
Canada	16.6*
France	19.5*
West Germany	19.4

Italy	24.1
Netherlands	14.0
Sweden	11.1
Switzerland	13.5
United Kingdom (England and Wales)	17.9
United States	20.7

* 1974 for these countries; see note 2 a.

The mean for the ten countries is 17.60. The standardized index shown in the first line of table 3-5 is obtained by dividing each country's perinatal mortality rate by 17.60 and rounding to two decimal places. Thus:

	Standardized Index for Perinatal Mortality
Australia	1.09
Canada	0.94
France	1.11
West Germany	1.10
Italy	1.37
Netherlands	0.80
Sweden	0.63
Switzerland	0.77
United Kingdom (England and Wales)	1.02
United States	1.18

A parallel calculation was done for the other sixteen age- and sex-specific mortality rates. For index A the index rates for all seventeen rates were then added for each country, divided by seventeen and rounded to two decimal places. Index B is similar except that the figures for perinatal and infant mortality were given three times the weighting of the other rates, on grounds of their greater relative significance in terms of lost lives and lost years of life. The differences in national rankings on index A and index B are minor: The first five countries are not affected, nor are the last two.

is more suited to micro analysis of particular conditions and services than to illustrations at the national level. But one must sound a warning to anyone who assumes too readily that health-care-expenditure increases can be halted without penalty to patients.

The United Kingdom provides the outstanding example among these ten countries of relatively low health-care expenditures over a long period, even taking into account its low GNP per capita (see, for example, figure 3-6).

Rates per 1,000 live births

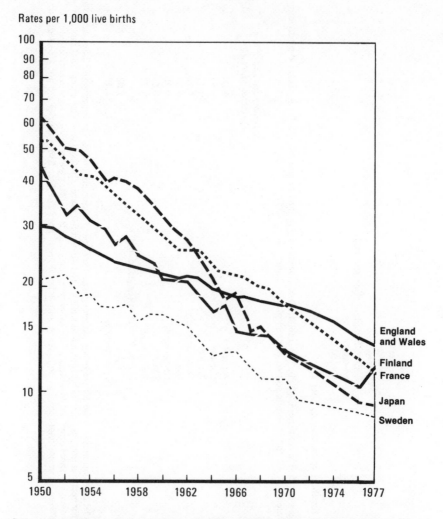

Source: Court Report, *Fit for the Future* (London: HMSO, 1976), Command 6684. Reprinted with permission, updated to 1976 from *On the State of the Public Health for the Year 1977* (London: HMSO), p. 23, table 1.12 and the corresponding publication for 1978, p. 20, table 1.11.

Figure 3-13. Infant Mortality Rates in Selected Countries, 1950-1977

Comparatively, British Ministers of Health have on the face of it had justification for their claims that the National Health Service is cost effective. But they have not had good grounds for complacency. The troublesome point in the United Kingdom's case is not its relative health status, which is moderately good (table 3-4). It is its comparatively slow rate of improvement relative to others, at least on some indicators. Infant mortality provides an example (figure 3-13). Many factors other than health expenditure may lie behind this. Nevertheless, death rates for the very young (under one week) have been affected by advances in medical care; and British mortality rates for this group give no grounds for complacency.

The main point, then, is simply to sound a warning to those who think primarily in terms of cost containment.

Finally, opportunities to obtain better value for money call for specific analysis of needs, and the cost and impact of feasible responses to them. Fashionable calls for prevention rather than treatment, for community care rather than institutional care, and for economy in the use of high-cost skills all contain an element of sense. But they are also far too simplistic because of the heterogeneity of health needs and the realities of what will actually work in a specific place at a particular time. This theme goes beyond the scope of the present study; it is nevertheless worth bearing in mind as we look in more detail at health-care expenditures in chapter 4 and return in chapter 5 to conclusions and implications. If there were a simple way of paying for health care, one that avoided both hardships to individuals and escalating costs, it would have been found long ago in one system or another. Useful steps forward are more likely to be aimed at some limited facet of the total problem, which should, however, be seen within the broader context, so that attempts to find solutions do not do more harm than good. It is one purpose of this book to provide such a context.

4

The Composition of Health-Care Expenditures

When countries document health-care spending in any detail, they tend to concentrate on government expenditures and to use a single set of headings, dictated by their own particular public-sector accounting conventions. But since the mix between public and private spending varies sharply from country to country, any worthwhile international comparison must consider both. Moreover, no single classification of expenditures, even one that was standardized between countries, could be as illuminating as a look at the figures from several complementary perspectives. This chapter therefore tries to analyze total spending in four different ways, by looking at: (1) where the money comes from; (2) who controls and administers the institutions and agencies through which it is spent; (3) what resources the money buys for use in health care; and (4) what health services are provided. A fifth expenditure classification—to whom the services are provided—is not adequately covered in this analysis, although some aspects of it are discussed in the fourth section, on services.

Who Pays: Sources of Finance

Health-care funding is either public or private in nature. Public funding includes such sources as general taxation (which may be central, regional, or local) and compulsory insurance. Private funding includes most voluntary insurance and all direct payments by consumers. Public-insurance schemes with a substantial element of direct public subsidy have been considered as public finance in this book, even though participation in them may not be compulsory.

Using these definitions, the proportion of total health-care expenditures covered by public sources ranged in 1975 from 42.7 percent to over 90 percent (see figure 4-1 and table 4-1). This proportion is a measure of the transfer of payment from the consumer to the community and thus of compulsory sharing of the burden of health-care financing. Of the ten countries the United States stood alone in 1975 in having less than half the total health-care bill paid publicly. At the other extreme, the United Kingdom, Sweden, and Italy were all overwhelmingly publicly financed. Among the remaining countries West Germany, France, and Canada were approximately three-quarters reliant on public finance; and Switzerland, the Netherlands, and Australia were two-thirds publicly financed.

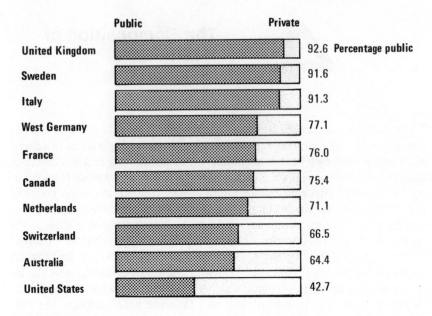

Source: Table 4-1.

Figure 4-1. Sources of Finance for Health-Care Expenditures: The Mix between Public and Private in 1975 as a Percentage of Total

Common to all the countries until now has been a tendency for the publicly financed share of total expenditure to rise with time, and the privately financed share to fall. The United States provides the best-documented example (figure 4-2). However, this trend is not irreversible. Indeed it is probable that there will soon be movement in the opposite direction, with governments increasingly determined (as remarked in chapter 3) to check further increases in public spending. In Australia, for example, the public proportion of health-care finance, which rose from the 64.4 percent shown in figure 4-1 to about 75 percent following the introduction of the Whitlam government's Medibank scheme on 1 July 1975, was cut back under the Liberals to around 66 percent.

The ways in which public finance for health care is raised follow two main patterns. The first is the use of general tax revenues, and the second is the use of some form of compulsory or subsidized health insurance (see figure 4-3). Five of the ten countries, comprising the four English-speaking countries and Sweden, use the first method predominantly. Switzerland falls into a category by itself: Although 63 percent of its public finance for health care is raised by taxation (particularly at the cantonal level), approximately one-quarter of this is then paid in subsidies to public-insurance

Table 4-1
Health-Care Expenditures by Source of Finance
(percentages of total expenditure)

	Australia (1974-1975 Fiscal)	Canada (1975)	France (1975)	West Germany (1975)	Italy (1975)	Netherlands (1974)	Sweden (1975)	Switzerland (1975)	United Kingdom (1974-1975 Fiscal)	United States (1974-1975 Fiscal)
1. Public										
a. General taxation (including subvention payments to public insurance schemes)	62.7	66.3	7.0	14.6	23.8	15.1	78.5	41.7	87.3	(31.0)
b. Public insurance	1.7	9.1	69.0	62.5	67.5	56.0	13.1	24.8	5.0	(11.7)
c. Other	—	—	—	—	—	—	—	—	0.3	—
d. Total public	64.4	75.4	76.0	77.1	91.3	71.1	91.6	66.5	92.6	42.7
2. Consumers										
a. Direct payment	21.1	19.5	19.6	12.5	8.7	27.3	8.4	33.5	5.8	27.1
b. Private insurance	13.8	2.5	3.0	5.3			—		1.2	25.6
c. Total consumers	34.9	22.0	22.6	17.8	8.7	27.3	8.4	33.5	7.0	52.7
3. Other	0.7	2.6	1.4	5.1	—	1.6	—	—	0.4	4.6
Total	100.0	100.0	100.0	100.0	100.0	100.0	100.0	100.0	100.0	100.0

Notes:

1. *Sources of data:* The sources are the national summaries for each country, with their supporting notes.

2. *Definitions:* General taxation is self-explanatory, but may be levied at many levels in the system (see text and national-summary notes). Public insurance mainly covers social security and similar compulsory schemes, but in Switzerland and the Netherlands includes publicly subsidized and regulated voluntary insurance. When general tax monies are channeled through public-insurance schemes by way of subsidies, they are assigned to the general-taxation category as the prime source. Public-insurance schemes are frequently related to employment, so that countries (such as France, Italy, and West Germany) with high proportions of the bill funded by public insurance rely heavily on statutory payments by employers and employees. Direct payments by consumers include payments for nonprescription drugs, except in the Netherlands. Private insurance is largely self-explanatory, and the figure given is subscription income rather than benefits paid. The difference from public insurance is that it is not compulsory, nor directly subsidized (although it may well be subsidized indirectly through tax deductibility of premiums). Like public insurance, it is frequently work-related, with part of the premiums paid by employers. The category "other" as a source of finance (number 3 in the table) comprises direct payments by employers (for example, in West Germany), and by philanthropic and voluntary organizations.

3. *Weaknesses in the data:* The table is reasonably complete and reliable. Some payments are known to be excluded in certain countries (see table 2-1 in the text). The breakdown between direct payment and private insurance is unknown for Italy, the Netherlands, and Switzerland, and is unreliable for several other countries (such as Canada), since direct payment is frequently calculated as a residual by deducting incomplete data on private health insurance.

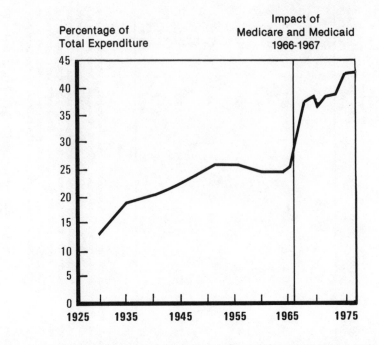

Source: DHEW, *Social Security Bulletin (Washington, D.C.: July 1978), table 1.*
Figure 4-2. United States: Public-Sector Share of Total Health-Care Expenditures

schemes. Australia has moved nearer to a social-security-insurance mode since the change of government from Labour to Liberal at the end of 1975. Italy, on the other hand, increased the general-taxation portion of public-health expenditure from 14 to 26 percent between 1974 and 1975 through a new public fund for general hospitals which is financed in part by social security and in part directly from the Treasury. This move in Italy was taken even further by the introduction of a national health service in January 1979. The ultimate intention is that this will be funded wholly from general tax revenues, and that the insurance funds will be dismantled.

Apart from these interesting recent changes by Australia and Italy, the mix between general-tax-revenue finance and compulsory insurance seems to depend more on history than on principle. Health services administered

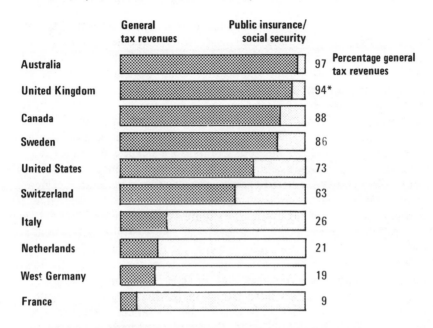

Figure 4-3. The Composition of Public Health-Care Expenditures in 1975

Source: Calculated from table 4-1.

Note: The United Kingdom figure is for fiscal 1974-1975. For 1975-1976 the percentage of general tax revenues dropped to 91 percent, with a corresponding increase in National Health Service contributions.

by government were originally financed from tax revenues in all these countries (including hospital services from a very early date in Sweden), whereas voluntary social-security schemes almost everywhere provided the initial means of spreading the cost of all other health services. These voluntary schemes later became compulsory (or subsidized and regulated) as governments sought to ensure coverage for those not yet included in them. The schemes have survived except where there has been a deliberate national change of policy away from them, as in the United Kingdom with the setting up of the National Health Service in 1948.

The contrasting merits of general tax revenue and compulsory-insurance financing can be argued. On the whole, the first is administratively simpler and cheaper, and should lead to health being considered on its merits alongside other public-expenditure programs. (The relatively low administrative cost of general-tax financing in part depends on the convention that tax collection is not charged out to health and other public-expenditure programs. This will be discussed further later in this chapter.) Compulsory-insurance schemes, on the other hand, may bring home more clearly to people (including employers and trade unions) the relationship between health services provided and their cost. But the choice between the two methods is far more important for the insurance industry, and for public policy on income distribution and taxation, than for health care or the level of health expenditures. Compulsory health insurance may, as in West Germany and the Netherlands, leave out top income earners; and it is normally less "progressive" (in a technical sense) in its impact on incomes.

More important for the health system, probably, is the centralization or decentralization of either method. Compulsory sickness insurance can be handled through a single centralized fund or through many small funds, more or less closely regulated. Taxation can similarly be central, regional, or local. Of the four countries using general tax revenues for more than 80 percent of their public-health finance (figure 4-3), the United Kingdom now uses entirely central as opposed to local tax, and Australia uses federal tax overwhelmingly. Provincial taxes account for more than half the total in Canada, taking the country as a whole (the richer the province, the lower the federal share, and vice versa), and the federal government has recently acted to change the open-ended nature of its financing commitment. In Sweden, on the other hand, 95 percent of the general tax revenue for health services is raised on a county rather than a national basis.

There is sufficient evidence from the United Kingdom and Canada to show that the fewer the sources of health-care finance, the tighter (for better and for worse) can be the control of health-care expenditures. The greater also, at least in theory, is the opportunity to equalize resources across the country as a whole. Conversely, the greater the dependence on a single powerful source of finance (whether central or provincial), the less may people perceive local freedom and responsibility to pay for the services that they want.

Turning from public to private sources of finance, the main sources are direct payment by consumers and payment by voluntary insurance, with direct provision by employers and philanthropic organizations as subsidiary sources, particularly in West Germany and the United States. The breakdown among these sources is not always available, but direct payment by consumers accounts for approximately one-fifth to one-quarter of total health-care expenditures in four countries (see figure 4-4). These figures include payments by consumers for nonprescription drugs. Such expenditures may or may not be a deliberate, planned element of national policy, and they may be borne by a larger or smaller proportion of consumers. In the United States they include payments (sometimes large ones) by those who are inadequately covered by voluntary insurance, and by the public schemes for the old and the poor. Major gaps in public and private health-insurance coverage for Americans in mid-1978 included (out of a total population of some 220 million) 24 million having no coverage whatsoever, 19 million having

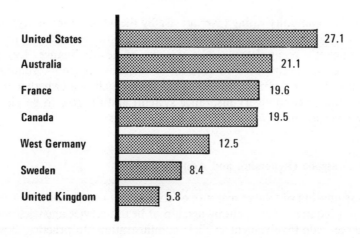

United States   27.1
Australia   21.1
France   19.6
Canada   19.5
West Germany   12.5
Sweden   8.4
United Kingdom   5.8

Source: Table 4-1.
Note: Information was not available for Italy, the Netherlands, and Switzerland.
Figure 4-4. Direct Payment by Consumers in 1975, Excluding Voluntary
Insurance (Percentage of Total Health-Care Expenditures)

inadequate coverage, and 88 million having no coverage for catastrophic incidents of sickness [37]. In France, on the other hand, the direct payments by consumers represent primarily a deliberate, planned element of national policy (the *ticket modérateur*) that most people should pay a proportion (usually one-quarter) of most minor health expenses. This, it is argued, is a way of moderating demand through the normal interplay of free-market forces, while shielding everyone from catastrophe. The difficulty is to pitch such charges at a level where they do restrain demand and provide worthwhile revenue, while at the same time not deterring people who need help. In view of mounting concern among governments about health-care costs, it seems inevitable that more countries will experiment with such schemes as the French *ticket modérateur*, involving cash payments by the user that may or may not be recoverable from a third-party payer at a later date. There remain the dangers of raising undesirable barriers to access and of increasing administrative complexity [38].

In summary, fairly comprehensive information on sources of finance is available. Countries fall into recognizable groups according to the mix between private and public sources, and between the reliance on general tax revenue and on compulsory, earmarked insurance. The trend everywhere until recently has been toward more reliance on public finance, and hence toward a *compulsory* spreading of the responsibility for meeting the costs of health care. This means not only that individuals are increasingly protected at the moment when they use health services, but also that the basis of protection is community rating (average use by the whole community), not individual risk. In this sense all the countries except the United States now have predominantly compulsory public systems of health finance. Key policy issues are the continuation or reversal of the move to public funding, the centralization or decentralization of the method chosen (whether this is a general-tax or compulsory-insurance system) and the role to be played by direct charges and *ticket modérateur* copayments.

Who Controls: Ownership and Administration

The assumption of a large measure of community responsibility for finance need not require government ownership of health-service agencies nor even any large-scale involvement in their administration. In practice, however, public regulation and intervention in any field tend to follow, sooner or later, on the heels of public finance. Few politicians and government administrators will stand aloof indefinitely from detailed intervention in the spending of large sums of public money, especially when some irregularity occurs or a public controversy arises. So it is not surprising that there is a correlation ($r = 0.652$) between reliance on public sources for health-care finance and the proportion of total expenditure spent in government-owned and -administered institutions (see figures 4-1, 4-5, and 4-6 and table 4-2).

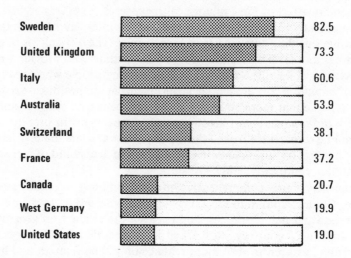

Sweden	82.5
United Kingdom	73.3
Italy	60.6
Australia	53.9
Switzerland	38.1
France	37.2
Canada	20.7
West Germany	19.9
United States	19.0

Source: Table 4-2.

Figure 4-5. Percentage of Total Health-Care Expenditures Spent in Government-Administered Institutions in 1975

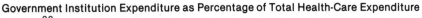

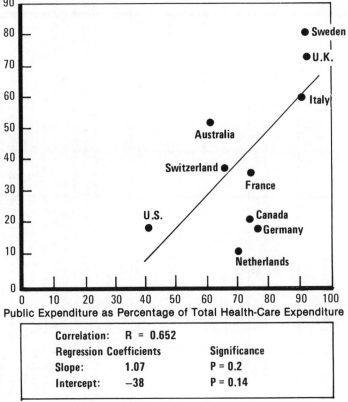

Source: Tables 4-1 and 4-2.

Figure 4-6. Government-Institution Expenditure as Percentage of Total Health-Care Expenditure by Public Expenditure as Percentage of Total Health-Care Expenditure

The boundaries between different types of ownership are not always clear cut, particularly when the reliance on public finance is high. For example, is a university that is funded overwhelmingly by government a government institution, or is it a nongovernment charitable undertaking? Even the boundary between nonprofit and for-profit institutions can be unclear, and some countries found it impossible to make this distinction with any confidence (table 4-2). Nevertheless, at another level the distinctions are important. In both the United Kingdom and Sweden, the two countries most reliant on public finance for health care, the issue of whether physicians are state employees or independent contractors to the state is an emotional

Table 4-2
Health-Care Expenditures by Ownership-Administration of Institutions
(percentages of total expenditure)

	Australia (1974-1975 Fiscal)	Canada (1975)	France (1975)	West Germany (1975)	Italy (1975)	Netherlands (1974)	Sweden (1975)	Switzerland (1975)	United Kingdom (1974-1975 Fiscal)	United States (1974-1975 Fiscal)
1. Government institutions	53.9	20.7	37.2	19.9	60.6	10.5	82.5	38.1	73.3	19.0
2. Non-government owned as nonprofit, such as charitable institutions	0-12.6	37.1	1.6-17.8	} 80.1	} 39.4	55.7	Negligible	14.6	Negligible	0-36.2
3. Private, for-profit institutions and contractors	33.5-46.1	42.2	44.7-60.9	} 80.1	} 39.4	33.8	17.5	47.3	26.7	44.8-81.0
4. Other			0.3							
Total	100.0	100.0	100.0	100.0	100.0	100.0	100.0	100.0	100.0	100.0

Notes:

1. *Sources of data*: The sources are the national summaries for each country, with their supporting notes.

2. *Definitions*: Government institutions include institutions and agencies owned and run by central, provincial, or local government, or (as in Italy) by the social-security system. This definition is unambiguous in many cases, but not in all. As mentioned in the text, universities and university hospitals are a case in point. They are nonprofit, but whether they are government or nongovernment can be disputed and may be viewed differently in different countries. The same applies to "voluntary" hospitals in several countries, if they are largely funded by government yet run by nongovernment boards. Thus there is a blurred boundary with the nongovernment, nonprofit sector. Similarly, the demarcation between profit and nonprofit can be unclear or at least may go unrecorded by government, as in West Germany and several other countries. Where possible I have defined, by analogy, a *minimum* size of the for-profit sector, including (for example) physicians and others in private practice or working as independent contractors, the pharmaceutical companies, and other medical suppliers. In three cases this left a grey area, which may be nonprofit or for-profit: I have expressed this by giving a minimum-to-maximum range for the for-profit sector in line 3 and (inversely) for the nonprofit sector in line 2.

3. *Weaknesses in the data*: As stated in note 2, there are definition problems at the margin between the sectors. Moreover estimation is necessary because national recording is typically less complete (even for public finance) on this facet than on the origin of the money (table 4-1). The data should therefore be taken not as precise but as indicative of the broad pattern in each country, and of *major* differences between countries.

one. In the United States the for-profit motivation of many operators in the nursing-home field (and increasingly in general hospitals also) is not identical with that of operators of nonprofit institutions. And in the Netherlands, which has a peculiar genius for overlaying older administrative forms without destroying them, small charitable foundations survive with a high degree of robust independence despite their almost total reliance on state funds.

It is perhaps surprising, and refreshing, to find that in no country is the degree of government ownership and administration as high as the reliance on public financing, and that in some countries, such as the Netherlands and Canada, it is much lower than one might expect.

The differentiation between public funding (table 4-1) and government ownership-administration seems well worth preserving. There are very good reasons, touched on in chapter 3, why the financing of health care and the control of resources flowing into the health system should be shared, communal concerns. Although there are grave difficulties about public funding of private institutions (apparent in France, Australia, and the United States, for example), the reasons for government to take over ownership and administration, particularly on a centralized basis, are less than overwhelming. Sheer size becomes a problem in any centralized health system, and governments are not skilled at running large, complex operations especially when (as in health services) administrative flexibility is needed at the local level. Moreover, as an ex-minister of health remarked [39], the attitude toward the shortcomings of a decentralized system is typically far more constructive, while a centralized one is filled with a deafening chorus of complaint about the ineptitude of the system.

Resources Used

It is much more difficult than it should be to obtain a breakdown of health-care expenditures in resource terms. Data is often available only for public hospitals, and by itself this is of little value for resource analysis without similar information for other hospitals and for services in the community. Moreover, classifications vary, especially in functions like laboratory analysis and equipment maintenance, which are sometimes carried out by private contractors and sometimes by employed staff. There seems, however, to be quite close correspondence among countries in the proportional shares of expenditure, so that a reasonable standard composition emerges (see figure 4-7 and table 4-3). These estimates include capital as well as current spending, and they attempt to break down expenditures in *all* services. Where possible, for example, gross fees paid to physicians have been allocated between personnel and nonpersonnel costs; and hospital

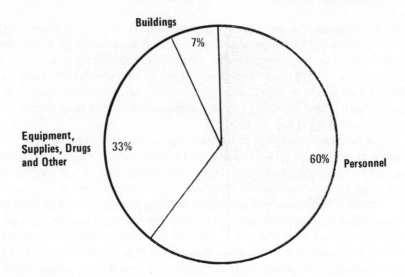

Source: Table 4-3.

Figure 4-7. Composition of Health-Care Expenditures in Resource Terms (Approximate Composite Picture)

drugs are included in drug costs along with pharmaceuticals purchased outside hospitals, with and without prescription.

Personnel

Salaries and wages are the largest single expense category, accounting in the seven countries for which data is available for 55 to 65 percent of total costs (see figure 4-8). The actual differences among countries are probably smaller than these figures suggest, owing to variations in the residual category (other costs) in table 4-3. If, for example, the manpower element in other costs is assumed to be similar to that in the bulk of health expenditures, then the Canadian and United Kingdom manpower percentages in figure 4-8 rise, respectively, to 64 and 62 percent. This proportion has held roughly constant over time, since expenditure on personnel has risen in line with total health-care spending. Increased salary and wage rates have been partly responsible, along with the moves toward equal pay for women and stronger union representation. Manpower numbers have also risen since, as noted in chapter 3, technological development in the health-care field seldom saves labor. Frequently, indeed, new forms of treatment, such as advanced forms of surgery and intensive care, require additional skilled people. Physician numbers, for which moderately reliable statistics are available, illustrate this point (see table 4-4).

Table 4-3
Health-Care Expenditures by Resource
(percentages of total expenditure)

	Australia (1974-1975 Fiscal)	Canada (1975)	France (1975)	West Germany (1975)	Italy (1975)	Netherlands (1974)	Sweden (1975)	Switzerland (1975)	United Kingdom (1974-1975 Fiscal)	United States (1974-1975 Fiscal)
1. Manpower										
a. Doctors (general practice)		7.1	7.8						5.3	
Doctors (all other)		10.8	9.5						5.9	
Doctors (total)		17.9	17.3		23.3	17.0			11.2	(17.5)
b. Dentists		5.0	7.7			5.0			2.2	
c. Nurses (qualified)					15.9				12.3	
Nurses (other)									7.9	
Nurses (total)		17.1	33.1						20.2	
d. Professional and technical		6.4			2.5				5.8	
e. Administrative, clerical, and auxiliary	63.2	8.8			15.2				18.4	
Total manpower		55.3	58.1		56.9		58.5	64.6	57.8	
2. Pharmaceuticals										
a. Prescribed	8.4	5.9	17.3	13.4	14.4	14.3	5.5		9.3	
b. OTC	4.9	4.5	3.7	4.5	5.6		3.5		3.4	
Total	13.3	10.4	21.0	17.9	20.0		9.0	8.5	12.7	
3. Buildings	7.0	5.2	19.5	4.6		7.4	7.0	7.0	7.1	> 8.3
4. Equipment and Supplies	16.5	13.4			23.1		25.5	19.9	15.4	3.8
5. Other		15.7	1.4	1.1					7.0	
Total	100.0	100.0	100.0	100.0	100.0	100.0	100.0	100.0	100.0	100.0

Table 4-3 *(continued)*

Notes:

1. *Sources of data:* The sources are the national summaries for each country, with their supporting data.

2. *Definitions: Manpower* expenditures are primarily salaries and wages, with associated costs such as superannuation. For independent contractors I have attempted to break down gross fees, so that (in the case of physicians) the cost allocated against physicians represents fees net of expenses, and expenses are allocated among expenditure heads. With respect to the definitions of different categories of personnel (such as professional and technical), see the notes to table 4-6. *Pharmaceutical* expenditures are divided between drugs supplied against prescription, including hospital drugs, and nonprescribed, over-the-counter drugs. In general, pharmaceutical expenditures are at retail prices, but hospital drugs present an inconsistency because they are usually recorded at cost, with associated salaries and wages classified under manpower. When this information is available, the *buildings* classification represents expenditure on new buildings and major renovation in the year in question. In some countries (particularly Italy and the Netherlands) such expenditure is mainly reimbursed via an amortization charge, rather than at the time when the expenditure is incurred. When this is the practice, the amortization charge has been included in the estimate of buildings expenditure. For most countries the expenditure recorded applies entirely or chiefly to hospitals, and spending on buildings for other purposes often goes unrecorded. In the private, for-profit sector, capital expenditure is frequently recovered through fees rather than direct or via an amortization charge. *Equipment and supplies* is intended to cover all medical and nonmedical items other than pharmaceuticals and major buildings work. The items cover a wide spectrum, and frequently expenditure on them can be derived only as a residual, after deducting other items. The heading *other*, where identified separately (as in Canada and the United Kingdom), applies to expenditure for which the resource breakdown is not known.

3. *Weaknesses in the data:* There are disappointing gaps, primarily because of incompleteness of recording in most countries. A resource breakdown and manpower numbers generally are available for the public hospitals, but not for private hospitals, nor (in many cases) for services outside hospital. Manpower expenditures, where given in table 4-3, should be reasonably reliable. Pharmaceutical costs are not complete in some cases; this problem is discussed in the section on pharmaceuticals of chapter 4 of this book. Buildings expenditure is also reported with varying completeness, as previously discussed in note 2. Since equipment and supplies is estimated largely as a residual, it should be treated with particular caution. There is also a conceptual problem in how far the analysis is taken: supplies (and particularly services provided on a contract basis) may well have a high manpower element in a resource analysis of the supplier's own costs.

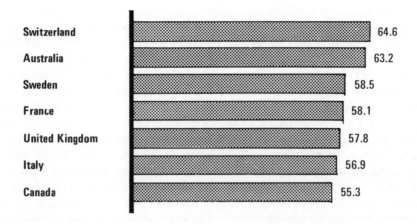

Switzerland	64.6
Australia	63.2
Sweden	58.5
France	58.1
United Kingdom	57.8
Italy	56.9
Canada	55.3

Source: Table 4-3.

Note: Information was not available for West Germany, the Netherlands, and the United States.

Figure 4-8. Percentage of Total Health-Care Expenditures (Including Capital) Spent on Manpower in 1975

Table 4-4
Growth in Physician Numbers

| Country | Physicians per 10,000 Population | | | Percentage Change, 1960 to 1975 |
	1960	1970	1975	
Sweden	9.5	13.6	17.1	+80
Canada	11.0	14.6	16.4	+49
France	10.0	13.2	14.6	+46
Switzerland	13.5	14.2	18.6	+38
Netherlands[a]	11.2	12.5	15.3	+37
Australia	11.7	12.6	15.2	+30
West Germany	14.9	17.2	19.2	+29
Italy[b]	15.9	18.1	19.9	+25
United Kingdom[c]	10.5	12.3	13.1	+25
United States	13.4	15.8	16.7	+25
Average	12.2	14.4	16.6	+38

Source: Table 4-5 and WHO *World Health Statistics Annuals*, (Geneva: World Health Organization) various years.

[a]For the Netherlands the table 4-5 figure (15.0) is for 1974. It is updated to 1975 from the national summary.

[b]The Italian figures, as presented in this table, include physicians practicing dentistry.

[c]U.K. data are for England and Wales. The latest figure is 1974, not 1975 (see the 1977 WHO *Annual*, vol. 3, p. 57). The ratio of 13.1 is substantially higher than mine for 1975 in table 4-5, which is based on Alan Maynard and Arthur Walker, *Doctor Manpower, 1975-2000* [Research Paper no. 4 for the Royal Commission on the National Health Service (London: HMSO, 1978)]. Although I believe that my figure is more likely to be correct, I have used the WHO figures in the present instance because they should be consistent over time.

The increase in numbers also applies to other personnel. Whereas in 1970 a composite international estimate of health-care personnel was 150 per 10,000 population (say 4 percent of the working population) a similar estimate for 1975 would be 175 (approaching 5 percent of the working population). In both years physicians accounted for roughly one-tenth of total health-care personnel (see table 4-5). The apparent variations among countries in total health manpower from 112.5 per 10,000 population in Italy to 218.6 in Switzerland, as shown in table 4-5 are in part the result of different definitions as well as the incompleteness of some of the data. The large number of part-time workers in the health field causes differences, since the counts for Canada and the United Kingdom are on the basis of whole-time equivalents, whereas several other countries record total numbers, regardless of hours worked. Titles also create difficulties, and the variations in nursing numbers (from 15 to 43 per 10,000 for qualified nurses, and from 38 to 105 for total nurses) are partly attributable to this cause. A "qualified nurse" is not the same in every country, still less is there a standard definition for an auxiliary nurse.

More important than the differences, however, is the fact that health services in countries such as these employ very large numbers of people; and relatively little attention has been given at the national level (at least until recently) to this highly important and expensive resource. Illustrative of the neglect is the lack of even the most elementary personnel statistics on a comprehensive basis in most of the ten countries. While there is now a general recognition of the impact of wage negotiation on health expenditures, other aspects of personnel management are still grossly neglected. For example, when the decision came to apply the brakes sharply to health-sector funding in Canada in the early 1970s, there was within months a complete, unplanned change in the market for many categories of health-service staff. Canadian provinces that had been actively recruiting nurses from overseas in 1972 and early 1973 found themselves unable to offer jobs to many of their own newly qualified nurses less than a year later.

Medical manpower represents a particularly crucial case, where the lack of foresight is (at least in retrospect) extraordinary. In the 1960s most developed countries expanded their medical schools sharply. This was an expansionist era in higher education, and medicine was a popular and heavily oversubscribed faculty. Universities and ministries of education therefore ratified increases in intakes of medical students with little, if any, consideration of the impact on health services of the consequential growth in numbers of doctors at work. Sweden, for example, forecast an almost threefold increase in physicians between 1970 and 1990 [40]. Then government policies changed, at least with respect to immigration. (Once medical-school expansions have taken place, they are very hard to undo.) Canada and Australia, which used to import doctors in substantial numbers, have now cut immigration to a trickle, and most of the ten countries face an im-

Table 4-5
Health-Care Expenditures by Resource
(manpower numbers per 10,000 population)

	Australia (1974-1975 Fiscal)	Canada (1975)	France (1975)	West Germany (1975)	Italy (1975)	Netherlands (1974)	Sweden (1975)	Switzerland (1975)	United Kingdom (1974-1975 Fiscal)	United States (1975)
Doctors										
General practice	6.0	5.7	9.1	10.5	7.2	3.5		3.7	4.5	2.5
All other	9.2	10.7	5.5	8.7	10.8	11.5		14.9	7.4	14.2
Total	15.2	16.4	14.6	19.2	18.0	15.0	17.1	18.6	11.9	16.7
Dentists	(3.0)	3.5	4.8	5.1	(1.9)	3.0	8.6	6.1	3.2	5.0
Nurses										
Qualified	(35.8)	42.0	37.2	37.1	15.3	32.2[a]	59.1		26.7	42.7
Other		44.7	7.7	6.2*	22.3	40.0*			44.8	62.7
Total		86.7	44.9	43.3**[b]	37.6	72.2*			71.5	105.4
Professional and technical		26.3	106.3	17.7**	10.6	19.3*			20.5	63.4**
Administrative, clerical, and auxiliary		46.8		39.5*	44.4	49.6*		218.6	55.4	
Total		179.7**	170.6	124.8**	112.5	159.1**			162.0	190.5**

Notes:

1. *Sources of data:* The sources are the national data summaries, with their supporting notes.

2. *Definitions: Doctors* and *dentists* are self-explanatory. The figure given for dentists in Italy is solely for physicians practicing dentistry. *Nurses* are, in this table, divided between qualified and other. Qualified nurses are those who hold a recognized nursing qualification, such as a nursing degree, state registration, state enrolment, or state license. Others include auxiliary and assistant nurses, and students. The boundary between "other nurses" and "auxiliary staff" depends on the titles used and certainly varies from place to place. *Professional and technical staff* include all those doing scientific and technical work, other than doctors and nurses, such as pharmacists, laboratory staff, physiotherapists and other remedial therapists, engineers, and computer staff. *Administrative, clerical, and auxiliary staff* constitute the balance.

3. *Weaknesses in the data:* Except for Canada, France, and the United Kingdom, the data are unsatisfactory. There are some difficulties of definition, for example, in comparability of nursing qualifications and titles and in allocation of people to one group or another at the margin. There is also the problem of part-time staff, although these figures are expressed as far as possible in full-time equivalents. But the main weaknesses at present are straightforward gaps in recording. Typically, there are detailed statistics on grades and numbers of staff in *public* hospitals, but little or no data about community health services and the private sector. From a resource analysis and planning viewpoint, this incomplete information is virtually without value. The other main data source, the population census, does not fill the gap because many of the supporting occupations (such as catering personnel or clerical staff) are not classified as specific to health services. In such instances there is no way of capturing information about them from the census, yet their numbers are substantial. The U.S. census does contain information on place of employment, as well as on occupation, but does not distinguish between part-time work and whole-time equivalents. For purposes of comparison, I have used the U.S. figure for those in health-related occupations only, while noting that it is incomplete.

a* = Hospital personnel only.

b** = Incomplete totals, since some of the constituent figures are for hospital personnel only or (in the case of the United States) for health-service occupations only.

Table 4-6
Manpower Numbers in the Health-Care Field (Approximate Composite Picture)

| | Personnel per 10,000 population | |
	1970	1975
Physicians	15	16.5
Nurses (fully qualified)	26	35
Dentists	4	4
Pharmacists	5	5
Supporting staff	100	114.5
Totals:	150	175

Sources: Table 4-5 and R. Maxwell, *Health Care: The Growing Dilemma* (New York: McKinsey and Company, 1975), figure 22. Reprinted with permission.

Note: The 1970 figures are based on a survey of twenty countries, which explains the small difference in physician numbers from the average in table 4-4. It also affects the comparability of the nursing numbers.

pending situation of physician oversupply. Canada, for example, allowed 1,147 foreign medical graduates to enter the country in 1973, a number approximately equal to the number of new graduates from Canadian medical schools in that year. By 1976 the number had been cut to 300 through a change in federal immigration policy. Not only is this oversupply a ludicrous waste of human skills and specialist training, threatening frustration for some of each country's most talented young people, but it also represents a severe economic threat. The direct costs of physicians, about one-sixth of total health costs at present, do not pose the problem. In the United Kingdom, for example, where physicians are paid less than in the other nine countries (not only absolutely but also relative to the average earnings of production workers within Britain; see table 4-7), a 50 percent increase in physician salaries would add only 5.5 percent to total expenditures. The economic threat lies more in the discretionary work generated by each physician, since decisions on what services patients should have depend very largely on the judgment of the physician whom they consult. It is therefore highly probable, without assuming any malign conspiracy, that if the number of physicians at work increases, total health-services activity and expenditure will also rise, although not necessarily in direct proportion. Of course, the change in activity may come in the mix of work, rather than in the quantity as measured by number of physician visits or inpatient days.

The point is not that medical or other health manpower should have been held to the 1970 level. It is that to expand numbers trained for these occupations without thought of their employment was irresponsible, and will prove expensive.

Table 4-7
Doctors' Income in Relation to GDP per Capita and Earned Income, 1974 or Near Date

Country	GDP per Capita	Ratio of Doctors' Income to: Compensation of Employees per Employee	Average Production Worker's Gross Earnings
Belgium			
Physicians and dentists	6.3	3.7	5.2
Pharmacists	6.0	3.6	4.9
Canada	6.8	5.0	4.8
Denmark (1973)	5.7	4.0	3.8
Finland (1970)	5.2	5.0	4.2
France	7.0	4.3	7.0
Germany (1973)	8.5	5.6	6.1
Ireland (1973)	7.6	3.7	3.5
Italy (1973)	9.5	4.3	6.8
Netherlands (1973)	10.2[a]	5.0	6.3
New Zealand			
Physicians	6.2	(4.0)	3.9
Dentists	4.9	(3.1)	3.1
Norway	3.4	2.4	2.4
Sweden	4.6	3.3	3.5
United Kingdom (1973)	4.5	3.3	2.7
United States			
Physicians	6.7	4.5	5.6
Dentists (1972)	5.6	3.3	4.1
Dispersion[b]	1.7	.8	1.4
Average[c]	6.2	3.9	4.4

Source: Organization for Economic Cooperation and Development, *Public Expenditure on Health* (July 1977), p. 24, table 9. See also p. 25, the passage concerning definitions and the problems of international comparisons. Reprinted with permission.
[a]If GDP per person employed were used as the basis for this comparison, this apparent difference from other countries would be considerably reduced.
[b]Measured by standard deviation.
[c]Geometric mean.

Pharmaceuticals

The second largest category of expense, from a resource viewpoint, is pharmaceuticals, representing from 8.5 to 21 percent of total health-care spending (figure 4-9). These figures include both prescribed drugs and pharmaceuticals sold without prescription (except for the Netherlands, for which only expenditure on prescribed drugs is known). Expressed in U.S. dollars per capita the variation is fourfold, from $29 in the United Kingdom to $114 in West Germany, with six of the countries falling in the $50-$68 range (table 4-8). As a percentage of gross national product, the range is

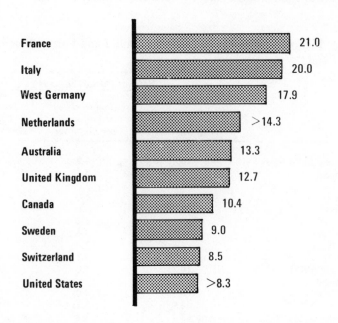

France　　　　　　　　21.0
Italy　　　　　　　　　20.0
West Germany　　　　 17.9
Netherlands　　　　　 >14.3
Australia　　　　　　 13.3
United Kingdom　　　 12.7
Canada　　　　　　　 10.4
Sweden　　　　　　　 9.0
Switzerland　　　　　 8.5
United States　　　　 >8.3

Source: Table 4-3.

Figure 4-9. Expenditure on Pharmaceuticals (Prescribed and OTC) as a Percentage of Total Health-Care Expenditures in 1975

from 0.59 in Switzerland to 1.68 in West Germany. The GNP figures can be compared for five countries with the recent European Economic Community (EEC) Report prepared by Abel-Smith and Grandjeat [10]. For France and the United Kingdom my figures and theirs are close. The difference for Italy can be explained by the incompleteness of my figure, which includes no estimate for hospital prescribing, since I was unable to obtain one. (My total costs for Italy do include hospital drugs, but they are not identified separately.) Conversely, for the Netherlands my figure is the more complete, since it does include an estimate of hospital prescribing, although both figures exclude over-the-counter (OTC) drugs. For West Germany I cannot explain the difference between the two estimates. Among the countries not covered by the EEC study, the estimate for the United States is incomplete, since most prescribed pharmaceuticals are excluded from the official American estimate for drugs, although included in total spending. The Swiss figures also are probably too low, owing to incompleteness of recording. Indeed, industry sources suggest that Swiss spending per capita on drugs lies between that of France and of Sweden. The true range is thus likely to be from approximately 0.75 percent of GNP in Canada, the United Kingdom, and Sweden, to more than twice that in West Germany, France, Italy, the Netherlands, and (probably) the United States.

Table 4-8

Expenditure on Pharmaceuticals (Prescribed and OTC) in 1975 in U.S. Dollars per Capita and as a Percentage of GNP

Country	Dollars per Capita	Percentage of GNP	(Percentage of GNP Given in EEC Report for Comparison)
West Germany	114.2	1.68	(1.40)
France	108.7	1.66	(1.70)
Netherlands	> 67.5	> 1.13	(> 0.80)
Sweden	64.5	0.77	
Australia	61.7	0.97	
Canada	52.8	0.74	
Switzerland	50.9	0.59	
United States	> 50.4	> 0.72	
Italy	44.8	1.43	(1.89)
United Kingdom	28.7	0.77	(0.75)

Sources: Calculated from tables 3-1 and 4-3.

Why do these differences exist? Logically, they must arise from variations either in the quantity and mix of drugs consumed, in the prices paid to the pharmaceutical companies, or in the methods and costs of distribution. That prices do vary is already documented [12], and it is unlikely to be coincidence that the three countries (Canada, the United Kingdom, and Sweden) with the lowest costs relative to GNP all have government-dominated systems of health funding (see, for example, figure 4-3) with an opportunity to use government influence in negotiating prices. It is also probable, although not yet documented, that differences in distribution patterns have a substantial impact on costs. Evidence on national consumption patterns is not comprehensive but is nevertheless sufficient to demonstrate that there are differences between countries that cannot be attributed to variations in morbidity [13]. Examples in 1971 included the very high use of phenylbutazone in Switzerland; the Swedish penchant for vitamins and tonics; and the French consumption of suppositories, medicines for the liver, and lactobacillus. National habit, one has to assume, plays an important part in the prescribing of drugs and the buying of drugs without prescription.

Buildings

Leaving aside the category of supplies and other, since it is too heterogeneous for useful comparison, the final resource category is buildings. Data is available for eight countries, and for five of these the variation is narrow, from 7 percent to roughly 7.5 percent (see table 4-9). The three countries that fall below 7 percent all have large elements of their

Table 4-9
Spending on Buildings as a Percentage of Total Health-Care Expenditures in 1975

Country	Percentage
Netherlands	7.4
United Kingdom	7.1
Australia	7.0
Sweden	7.0
Switzerland	7.0
Canada	5.2
West Germany	4.6
United States	3.8

Source: Table 4-3.
Note: Information not separately available for France and Italy.

system administered by institutions outside government, which probably recover much of their capital costs through their prices for services (see figure 4-5). Most of this expenditure is on hospital buildings, principally on construction and major renovation. Maintenance expenditure and minor alterations that are carried out by employed staff are likely to be included under personnel rather than under buildings. Equipment should be included in equipment, supplies, and other.

Comparative analysis of hospital expenditure belongs more properly in the next section, dealing with spending by service. Buildings themselves vary greatly in age and condition among and within the ten countries, depending on when the major expansions of hospital services took place in the past, and on the relative tightness or generosity of budgets more recently. When money is tight this category of expenditure is (within the constraints imposed by contracts already awarded) cut back more sharply than running expenses. For example, in Sweden from 1971 to 1974 the county councils and local authorities were forbidden to raise taxes, and the central government also sought to reduce its own spending, with a restraining effect on the growth of health expenditures as a whole and a disproportionate effect on capital expenditure (see table 4-10).

Fiscally, this is easy to understand. When cuts must be made, the treasury axe falls wherever cuts are in fact possible, and it is clearly easier to postpone the start of new buildings than to fire employees. The long-term effect on the health sector is another matter, although it must be said that old buildings are not always a handicap. They are usually very solidly constructed and less dependent on sophisticated, fallible engineering and maintenance services than modern replacements. They act as a straitjacket only when they stand in the way of long-overdue changes in treatment and living patterns as, for example, with many of the large psychiatric hospitals

Table 4-10
Health-Care Expenditures in Sweden

	1970	1971	1972	1973	1974	1975
Total health-care expenditures (milion kronor)	12,681	14,491	15,833	17,082	20,070	24,396
Percentage of GDP/GNP spent on health care	7.4	7.9	8.0	7.8	8.1	8.5
Capital spending (million kronor) State	222.4	156.7	227.5	160.1	194.3	207.6
Counties and county boroughs	1,461.9	1,404.0	1,277.7	1,206.5	1,316.7	1,678.5
Total	1,684.3	1,560.7	1,505.2	1,366.6	1,511.0	1,866.1
Total public capital ÷ Total expenditures from all sources × 100	13.3	10.8	9.5	8.0	7.5	7.6

Source: Statistika Centralbyrån, Stockholm, for lines 1 and 2; *Public Health in Sweden 1975*, (Stockholm: National Board of Health and Welfare, 1977) p. 70, table C3 for capital spending.

built a century ago, or in some instances with the siting and configuration of general hospitals. Buildings are primarily important as shells that enable or contrain the activities within them.

Postscript on Resources

A resource analysis of health-care expenditures leads to an essentially simple conclusion. To control health-care expenditures one must control manpower (numbers and wage rates); pharmaceuticals (prices and distribution costs, prescribing patterns, and brand availability); spending on buildings and major equipment; and numbers of institutional places. All this, however, says nothing about effectiveness.

Services Provided

Comparisons of expenditure by service are seriously impeded by accounting differences. Taking hospital expenditure first, accounting practice varies among countries in two important ways, as summarized in table 2-1 (item 11). First, fees paid to physicians for attending hospitalized patients may be included in hospital costs or excluded from them. If excluded, they are lumped with physicians' fees for care outside hospitals. Second, hospital-based outpatient care may be classified with other ambulatory care or with inpatient treatment, and only rarely is its cost separately identified. Furthermore, as noted in item 3 of table 2-1, there are also important differences in the boundary between hospitals and other caring institutions such as nursing homes and residential homes for the elderly.

In view of these major classification problems, apparent differences must be viewed with caution. For hospital services, it seems best to differentiate three groups of countries according to their different methods of classifying costs, and to make comparisons primarily within rather than between groups (tables 4-11 and 4-12). These figures for hospital expenditure can also be expressed as percentages of GNP (table 4-13). That Sweden's figures for hospital spending are so high in tables 4-11 and 4-13 is not surprising: It has the most hospital-dominated health system of the ten countries, with more than 150 hospital beds per 10,000 population and with well above average rates for hospital admissions and days of hospitalization per capita (see table 4-14). Also, within group A, Sweden and the United Kingdom have more extensive hospital-based ambulatory care than do Switzerland and Italy, which helps to explain their higher hospital percentages in table 4-11. The most puzzling figures are those for West Germany, which are the lowest for hospital care as a percentage of total expenditure

Table 4-11
Hospital Expenditure as a Percentage of Total Health-Care Expenditures in 1975

Country	A All-inclusive Costs Group	B Mixed Group	C Costs Exclusive of Private Physicians' Fees and Expenditures on Hospital-Based Ambulatory Care
Sweden	71		
United Kingdom	63		
Canada	59		
Australia		57	
Netherlands		53	
United States		50	
Italy	48		
Switzerland	45		
France			38
West Germany			35
Group averages	57	53.5	36.5

Sources: Tables 2-1 and 4-12 and national summaries.
Note: Group A includes associated physicians' costs and expenditure on outpatient departments in hospital expenditures. Group B excludes the fees of private attending physicians but includes hospital-based ambulatory care. Group C excludes both items.

Table 4-12
Health-Care Expenditures by Service
(percentages of total expenditure)

	Australia (1974-1975 Fiscal)	Canada (1975)	France (1975)	West Germany (1975)	Italy (1975)	Netherlands (1974)	Sweden (1975)	Switzerland (1975)	United Kingdom (1974-1975 Fiscal)	United States (1974-1975 Fiscal)
1. Hospitals										
a. Current excluding amortization										
Inpatient	43.6	53.8		31.5		45.2	64.1	37.9	56.9	46.6
Outpatient	7.4			NA						
b. Capital	5.9	5.2		3.5		7.4	7.0	7.0	5.9	3.8
c. Total	56.9	59.0	38.0	35.0	48.0	52.6	71.1	44.9	62.8	50.4
2. Care outside hospitals										
a. Primary care	30.0	18.5							20.8	
b. Specialist care		9.1							—	
c. Capital	1.1	NA							0.5	
d. Total	31.1	27.6	44.5	30.2	34.9	41.9	24.6	41.0	21.3	40.0
3. Self-medication	4.9	4.5	3.8	4.5	5.6	Excluded	3.5	5.0	3.2	
4. Other services										
a. Public health	3.1	3.2	1.1	3.2	2.2	1.1	NA	3.8	6.2	2.4
b. Research	0.5	1.1	1.1	0.3	NA	Largely excluded	0.4	5.3	1.5	2.5
c. Education	1.4	Largely excluded	1.2	1.7	NA	NA	Largely excluded		NA	Largely excluded
d. Other	—		—	19.1	2.9	—	—	—	—	—
e. Total	5.0	4.3	3.4	24.3	5.1	1.1	0.4	9.1	7.7	4.9
5. Administration	2.1	1.7	9.3	6.0	6.4	4.4	0.4	NA	0.9	4.7
6. Other	—	2.9	1.0	—	—	—	—	—	4.1	—
Total	100.0	100.0	100.0	100.0	100.0	100.0	100.0	100.0	100.0	100.0

Table 4-12 *(continued)*

Notes:

NA = Not separately available but included elsewhere.

1. *Sources of data:* The sources are the national data summaries, with their supporting notes.

2. *Definitions:* As shown in table 2-1 (item 11) and discussed in chapter 3, accounting practice varies among countries in the definition of *hospital current expenditure.* In France and West Germany, it excludes fees paid to private physicians for attending patients in the hospital and also excludes the cost of hospital-based ambulatory care. In Australia, the Netherlands, and the United States it similarly excludes private physicians' fees, but includes hospital ambulatory care. In the remaining five countries it includes both items. There is also a boundary problem between hospital expenditure and other institutional care. Where there is a substantial nursing-home sector, as in the United States, Canada, and the Netherlands, I have included it with hospital expenditure in this analysis. The amounts concerned can be identified separately in the national summaries. *Hospital capital expenditure* is based either on actual spending for new buildings and major renovation or (particularly in Italy and the Netherlands) on amortization (see item 4 in table 2-1). Except in the United States, there should not be double counting between the two methods. *Care outside hospitals* covers fees for service by physicians, dentists, and so on, and associated prescribing costs. For the countries previously mentioned, it includes elements of hospital-associated costs—those for attending physicians and for hospital-based outpatient activities. *Self-medication* concerns purchases of nonprescribed drugs, over the counter. This expense is not known for the Netherlands and, as explained in table 2-1 and chapter 2, is excluded from the Dutch total for health expenditure. For the United States the figure is not separately identifiable but is included. Under *other services, public health* typically comprises environmental and preventive activities, such as inspection of food premises, port health, and monitoring for environmental hazards. In some cases it also includes some child-health and immunization programs. Clearly, from the variation of expenditure under this heading, the scope of public health varies widely among countries. Laws and customs differ as to the range and scale of activities that governments undertake in this field, including whether the relevant public agencies are confined to a diagnostic role or themselves treat the individuals. Some overlap is likely with care outside hospitals (for child health and immunization) and (in the case of Germany) with item 4d in the table; moreover, certain countries (such as Canada) may well undertake health-education programs under this heading on a scale not yet attempted elsewhere. *Research* covers all medical and health-services research, wherever undertaken, except for pharmaceutical and similar research programs conducted by commercial companies and financed through product pricing. In most cases, recorded expenditure for research is incomplete, since some research is inseparable from service activities (although included within total costs), whereas some is financed from many dispersed sources, such as charitable donations (which may not be recorded at all within health-care expenditures). Item 4d under other services is primarily important for Germany, where it comprises:

	Percentage of Total Health-Care Expenditure
Diagnosis and surveillance	5.5
Rehabilitation services	2.0
False teeth	6.6
Spa treatment	5.0
	19.1

Arguably the first of these could be included under 4a, public health, but there could also be an element of primary care in it. There are aspects of all four items that fall outside the scope of health services in at least some of the other countries. The heading *administration* normally covers the costs of collecting and disbursing health-insurance monies (but not of collecting general taxation), and of running government health departments and agencies; the administration costs of individual hospitals are included in total health-care spending via hospital current expenditure (item 1a in the table). Finally, item 6 in the table refers to residual expenditure for which no breakdown by service is available.

3. *Weaknesses in the data*: The differing definitions of hospital expenditure (including or excluding attending physicians' fees and outpatient activities) provide a tiresome problem, since they mean that comparisons must be made primarily between countries using the same definition, rather than among all ten countries. Care outside hospital represents almost the reciprocal of this problem, since it normally includes the elements that are excluded by some national definitions from hospital expenditure. Nevertheless, something can be learned about each health system by understanding what accounting conventions it follows, and why, in classifying expenditure by service. The same can be said about most of the other headings: public health, research, education, and administration. The definitions do vary, and one should therefore be very cautious in drawing conclusions from the comparisons; but the variations in definition are well worth probing for the insights they give into the workings of each of the national systems.

Table 4-13
Hospital Expenditure as a Percentage of GNP in 1975

Group A (table 4-11)	
Sweden	6.0
United Kingdom	3.8
Canada	4.2
Italy	3.4
Switzerland	3.1
Group B	
Australia	4.2
Netherlands	4.2
United States	4.4
Group C	
France	3.0
West Germany	3.3

Sources: Tables 3-1 and 4-11.

despite the high level of hospital utilization shown in table 4-14. The explanation must lie with several factors rather than with a single one. Differences in definition (table 4-11) are partly responsible; as must also be the high element of German costs that lie outside hospitals, particularly physicians' offices, diagnosis and surveillance, rehabilitation, and spa treatment. Finally, lengths of stay are very long in German hospitals, and the lower intensity of care may be reflected in lower staffing levels (for example, fewer nurses) and hence in lower hospital costs. Incidentally, Hauser and Koch in their recent study [11] found a similarly low figure (36 pecent) for hospital care in Germany as a percentage of total expenditure.

The proportion of expenditures accounted for by personal care outside hospitals varies (figure 4-10) from 21.5 to 44.5 percent, countries ranking in approximately the reverse order from those in table 4-11. In other words, all other expenditures (public health, research, education, administration, and self-medication) do not vary greatly in the aggregate as a proportion of total health-care spending. It has recently been fashionable public policy in several of these countries to promote initiatives in community care. Whether this is sensible depends, naturally enough, on the appropriateness and cost effectiveness of the programs concerned. Since most episodes of illness do not call for highly skilled attention nor for expensive resources, it makes sense to hold these skills and resources in reserve. The cost effectiveness of health care in any country depends on the extent to which avoidable illness is prevented, and on the appropriateness of the matching of services to levels of health problems. Crucial variables within community-care programs, therefore, are how effectively and economically they are linked with preventive and self-care programs on the one hand, and with specialist referral services on the other.

Table 4-14
Summarized Hospital Statistics

	Hospital Beds per 10,000 Population	Hospital Admissions or Discharges per 10,000 Population	Days of Hospitalization per Capita
Group A (table 4-8)			
Sweden	152.4	1,811	4.7
United Kingdom	89.3	1,151	2.7
Canada	92.0	1,717	2.7
Italy	104.9	1,661	3.0
Switzerland	113.9	NA	NA
Group B			
Australia	123.9	1,900	2.4
Netherlands	101.4	1,028	2.3
United States	65.6	1,712	1.8
Group C			
France	102.4	1,613	3.4
West Germany	118.0	1,616	3.6

Sources: WHO *World Health Statistics Annual 1977* Volume III, supplemented as shown in the notes below. Unfortunately there are almost certainly some inconsistencies in the statistics, for example in the treatment of nursing home beds and of places for the mentally handicapped. NA = Not available.

Notes:

1. U.K. totals are basically for 1974, but include Scotland for 1975.

2. Figures for Italy were supplied by Istituto per la ricerca di Economia Sanitaria, except for days of hospitalization per head, which are from WHO and are for 1972.

3. Swiss beds are from WHO for 1971.

4. Australian beds are from WHO for 1972; they appear high relative to other sources. Admissions and days of hospitalization are estimated from J.S. Deeble, *Health Expenditure in Australia, 1960-61 to 1975-76*, (Canberra, ANC, 1978) tables 11 and 12.

5. Netherlands beds are for 1973 and are derived from *International Comparisons of Health Needs and Health Services* (London: McKinsey and Company, 1978). Admissions and days of hospitalization are from WHO and are incomplete.

6. U.S. figures are for 1975.

7. French figures are for 1973 and are from McKinsey and Company (see note 5).

8. Figures for West Germany are for 1975.

Perhaps the most important single strength of the British National Health Service is the pattern of general practice and the convention of referral from primary and secondary to tertiary care. Standards of general practice unfortunately vary, but when they are good the system works well and leads to an appropriate matching of levels of sophistication and cost to levels of problem. Over 80 percent of episodes of illness reaching the National Health Service are dealt with from start to finish by general practitioners who account, with associated prescribing costs, for well under 20 percent of total expenditure (see, for example, figure 4-11).

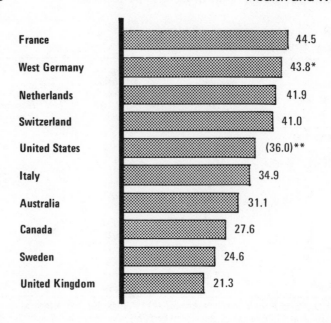

France	44.5
West Germany	43.8*
Netherlands	41.9
Switzerland	41.0
United States	(36.0)**
Italy	34.9
Australia	31.1
Canada	27.6
Sweden	24.6
United Kingdom	21.3

Source: Table 4-12.

Notes: The figure for West Germany includes expenditure on false teeth, rehabilitation services, and spa treatment from "other services" in table 4-12. The figure for the United States was obtained by estimating for self-medication.

Figure 4-10. Expenditure on Specialist and Primary Care Outside Hospitals as a Percentage of Total Health-Care Expenditure (1975)

The situation in the Netherlands is similar (as it also is, incidentally, in Denmark). In both countries the patient must normally be referred to a specialist by the general practitioner as primary-care physician. This control over access to the specialist, and the avoidance as far as possible of duplicated work-up between community-based and hospital-based specialists, may well be a key variable in the cost of the whole health-care system. Among the ten countries three different patterns prevail concerning access to specialists, with the highest-cost countries all allowing direct access to specialists (table 4-15). One can of course dispute which of these two variables is cause and which effect.

Another, and an increasingly important, variable is the way in which resources are matched to the needs of the elderly. Those over 65 represent only 8.5-15 percent of the total population in the ten countries, including a mere 3-5.5 percent for those over 75 (see table 4-16). But, as illustrated in figure 3-11, health-care spending rises steeply with age, so that the elderly—particularly those over 75—have a major impact on expenditures. This impact is felt in every general and psychiatric hospital and in primary

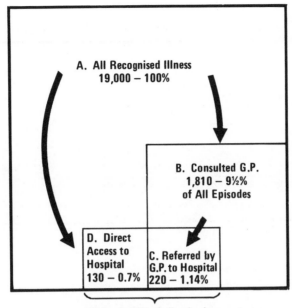

A. All Recognised Illness
19,000 – 100%

B. Consulted G.P.
1,810 – 9½%
of All Episodes

D. Direct
Access to
Hospital
130 – 0.7%

C. Referred by
G.P. to Hospital
220 – 1.14%

350 – 1.84% of all episodes
(18 percent of what reaches the Health Service)

Source: D. Crombie, "Changes in Patterns of Recorded Morbidity," in *Benefits and Risks in Medical Care*, edited by D. Taylor, p. 24, figure 1 (London: Office of Health Economics, 1974). Crombie's calculation is based on the Second National Morbidity Survey, 1970-1971 and (for total episodes) on M.E.J. Wadsworth, W.J.H. Butterfield, and R. Blaney, Health and Sickness: The Choice of Treatment (London: Tavistock, 1971). Reprinted with permission.

Figure 4-11. Thresholds of Awareness and Consultation (Episodes of Illness during Period of Study per 1,000 Patients at Risk)

care, as well as in programs specifically for older people. Thus, taking Great Britain as an example, in 1970 48 percent of general-hospital beds (excluding maternity and psychiatric beds) and 44 percent of mental-illness beds were occupied by patients over 65 (*Social Trends* 1973, p. 30, tables XIX and XXI). However, these 157,000 elderly patients represented less than 2.5 percent of the total number of elderly people in Great Britain at that time. Even adding a further 3 percent (see *Social Trends* 1979, p. 63, table 3.10) for those resident in old people's homes and other institutions, the total network of institutional provision is at present caring for no more than 6 percent of those over 65 [41]. The other 94 percent are living, with some degree of support, in the community. Thus, a relatively small reduction (say 1 in 35) in the proportion of the elderly able and willing to live at home would require a 50 percent increase in the hospital beds and institu-

Table 4-15
Access to Specialist Physicians and the Cost of Health Care

	Percentage of GNP Spent on Health Care
Countries with direct uncontrolled access by the patient to the specialist	
West Germany	9.4
United States	8.7
Sweden	8.5
France	7.9
Countries with direct access to specialists, but where patients will have to pay the difference between the specialist and general-practitioner rates of fee	
Australia	7.3
Canada	7.1
Italy	7.1
Switzerland	6.9
Countries where access to the specialist is normally by referral from the primary-care physician	
Netherlands	7.9[a]
United Kingdom	6.1

Sources: Chiefly J.G. Simanis *National Health Systems in Eight Countries* (Washington, D.C.: DHEW, 1975), for referral patterns, supplemented by my own enquiries in the countries concerned.

[a]Why, then, is the Netherlands' expenditure on health care comparatively high? Two major reasons are prosperity (relative to the United Kingdom) and lack of effective control over costs. Another interesting point is that methods of paying physicians may make a major difference. In the Netherlands the general practitioner is essentially salaried, and the specialist works on a fee-for-service basis. There is therefore a greater incentive to refer time-consuming cases than in the United Kingdom, where the specialist is salaried and the general practitioner receives fees for at least some services.

tional places required for older people. The position is basically similar in other survey countries, despite variations in the proportions of the elderly at present in hospitals and homes (table 4-17). In addition to the estimates in this table, the United States seems to fall in the upper half of the range shown, with 5 percent in long-term-care beds, plus the elderly in acute-care beds [43]. For Sweden the proportion of those over 65 in institutional care appears to exceed 12.5 percent [44], reinforcing the impression that of all the countries in this study Sweden is the most heavily dependent on institutional provision.

The percentage of old people in institutional care rises steeply with age and varies with marital status, financial position, and social and educational background. People living on their own, with low incomes and

Table 4-16
The Elderly Relative to Total Population, 1974

	Percentages of Total Population		
Country	65-74	75+	Total 65 and Over
Sweden	9.4	5.5	14.9
United Kingdom (England and Wales)	9.0	5.0	14.0
West Germany	9.4*	4.5*	13.9*
France	8.4*	5.2*	13.6*
Switzerland	7.9	4.2	12.1
Italy	7.8	4.0	11.8
Netherlands	6.7	3.9	10.6
United States	6.4	3.9	10.3
Canada	5.2	3.2	8.4
Australia	5.4*	3.0*	8.4*

Source: *International Comparisons of Health Needs and Health Services*, memorandum submitted to the Royal Commission on the National Health Service by McKinsey and Company, 1978.
Note: * = 1973.

limited education, are much more likely to be in homes or hospitals than are those with companions, with some financial means, and with higher educational attainment [42]. Yet substantial numbers of those living in private households live alone (30 percent in England), many have low incomes, and many (nearly 60 percent in England) suffer from some disability, the percentage increasing with age. Since the numbers and percentages of those over 75 are still increasing in the countries studied, the need for help at home and for institutional care will continue to rise for some time.

Table 4-17
The Elderly and Institutional Care

Country	Number of People Aged 65 and Over (1975)	Number in Institutional Care	Percentage in Institutional Care
Canada	1,938,100	186,790	9.6
Switzerland	775,600	c. 50,000	c. 6.5
England	6,496,000	c. 390,000	c. 6.0
West Germany	8,594,000	c. 344,000	c. 4.0
France	7,167,000	272,400	3.8

Sources (Canada): Health and Welfare Canada, Health Economics and Data Analysis Branch; (Switzerland and West Germany): *Die Altersfragen in der Schweiz* (Bern: Kommission für Altersfragen, 1967); (England): Audrey Hunt, *The Elderly at Home* (London: Office of Population, Censuses and Surveys, HMSO, 1978) para 3.1; (France): *Les personnes âgées vivant en institution* (Paris: CREDOC, 1977), p. III.

Moreover, it seems likely that the community will become more, rather than less, dependent on the support of institutional and other organized services for the elderly. The challenge presented to health and social services is great, not merely in terms of expenditure but also of developing responses that are truly appropriate in human terms.

Other aspects of expenditure by service can be dealt with very briefly. The proportion of total expenditure spent on self-medication—essentially the purchase of drugs over the counter, without prescription—varies from roughly 3 to 5.5 percent (table 4-18). (There is, of course, much more to self-care than self-medication. Diet, exercise, and life style all have far more impact on health than do drugs bought over the counter.)

Public-health services take from 1 to 6 percent of expenditures, the difference probably lying primarily in definition, particularly between public health and community care. Of the eight countries for which public-health expenditure is known, five record figures between approximately 2.5 and 4 percent; and this is probably a reasonable guideline figure, subject to closer scrutiny of what is covered by public health in each specific case.

Expenditures on education and research are low everywhere. Undoubtedly there is substantial underrecording of educational expenditure because it is not easy to draw the line between education and service; also, most countries fund at least part of their educational expenditures from their education budgets, rather than from those for health. Research expenditure is generally 1 percent or less of total expenditure (but 2.5 percent in the United States, which for many years gave medical research a high national priority [45]). Research by the pharmaceutical companies is additional to this figure, its cost being covered by pharmaceutical prices. When total health-care expenditures are under pressure, research tends to be squeezed, since it is less urgent than service. Many physicians combine a teaching, research, and service role; and in times of financial stringency

Table 4-18
Self-Medication as a Percentage of Total Health-Care Expenditures, 1975

Country	Percentage
Italy	5.6
Switzerland	5.0
Australia	4.9
Canada	4.5
West Germany	4.5
France	3.8
Sweden	3.5
United Kingdom	3.2

Source: Table 4-12.
Note: Data not available for the Netherlands and the United States.

their research time is the first to be eroded. But given the many unknowns in medical science and in health-care effectiveness, further squeezing of research should be challenged. One percent of total spending is a small investment, provided the research is well conceived and conducted, compared with the impact that answers to some of the unknowns could have.

Administration costs are underrecorded as a separate category in table 4-12 and in the underlying summaries, since on the whole the management costs for hospitals and other agencies are included with the costs of the service concerned and are not separately identified. The United Kingdom, for example, shows administrative costs of 0.9 percent in the table, reflecting the costs of central administration and of private health insurance; however, a more comprehensive estimate of 5.25 percent includes the administrative costs of the regions, areas, and districts. Most countries include the costs of their ministries of health, but Germany and Switzerland do not. None includes the costs of other ministries, and this exclusion is particularly important in the case of the countries that are most dependent on general-tax financing of their health-care systems (see figure 4-3). These qualifications must be borne in mind in considering the variation among countries from 0.4 to 9.3 percent in recorded administrative costs.

The convention that no costs of general-tax collection are attributed to health or other programs is one obvious reason that countries that use insurance methods have higher recorded administrative costs (see figure 4-12, $r = 0.8527$). Nevertheless, different accounting conventions are not the whole story; insurance modes of financing, whatever their merits, do add substantially to administrative costs.

Apart from calling attention to some differences between countries, this analysis of the composition of health-care expenditures in the ten countries identifies the key components that they share. These components—such as manpower numbers (particularly physicians), the balance between primary care and other referral services, and the range of support provided for the elderly—are the ones to which total expenditures are most sensitive.

In concluding this chapter, however, the supereminent importance of the client facet of expenditures must be emphasized—who the money is spent on and with what effect. We know very little about this, and it could not be covered adequately in this study. It is probably legitimate to hypothesize that spending levels strongly influence the levels of ascertainment of need and of service provision; and there is interesting recent evidence that this is indeed so in the field of chronic renal failure, where there is a correlation of roughly 0.8 between per-capita GNP and the number of renal patients on dialysis or with a functioning transplant (see figure 4-13). End-stage renal failure provides an important case study of the interrelationship between expenditure and service levels. In the United Kingdom, with its relatively tight system of health-care-expenditure control

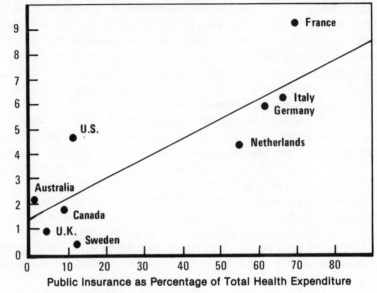

Correlation: R = 0.853
Regression Coefficients   Significance
Slope: 0.085   P < 0.002
Intercept: 1.20   P = 0.1

Source: Tables 4-1 and 4-12.

Figure 4-12. Administrative Expenditure as Percentage of Total Health-Care Expenditure by Public Insurance as Percentage of Total Health-Care Expenditure

and resource rationing, provision for end-stage renal failure is markedly different from that in most West European countries and the United States [46]. The United Kingdom, which was the first country to establish a national network of treatment centers, has fewer such centers per 1 million population than any other country in Western Europe except Portugal. Its program is much more heavily weighted toward home dialysis than any other, with a relatively high level of transplantation and a very low level of hospital dialysis. This probably makes it a highly cost-effective program, but people over about 50 with end-stage renal failure are far less likely to be accepted for treatment in the United Kingdom than in West Ger-

Renal patients (alive on dialysis or with a
functioning transplant) per million population

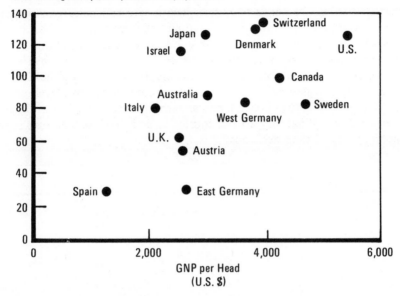

Source: A. J. Wing, *"Prospects for the Treatment of Renal Diseases,"* British Medical Journal, 1 October 1977. Reprinted with permission.

Figure 4-13.   Relationship between Number of Renal Patients at 31 December 1975 and GNP per Capita

many, France, Italy, or the United States [46]. The choice of whom to treat and whom not to treat is, of course, a very hard one in ethical and human terms. Too much medical intervention is a real hazard when resource constraints are not apparent, and treatment can then become inhumane [47]. Each country's choices may or may not be justifiable in light of human needs, the potential for treatment and the resources available. Presumably a much poorer country might not have any provision at all for end-stage renal failure; and that decision, although harsh, might be correct in its context. What is apparent, however, is that resource constraints have influenced the pattern of provision for end-stage renal failure in the United Kingdom. The choices made seem logical within the resource constraints. If more resources could be made available for the National Health Service as a whole and hence for the renal program, the choices would probably be different and older people would have a greater chance of treatment than they do at present. If resources were less, service levels would have to be reduced.

Were better information available, the interrelationship between expenditure levels and levels of provision would undoubtedly be paralleled in other specialties. Decisions to restrict health-care expenditures ultimately involve curtailing or withholding treatment for important human conditions. On the other hand, there is also good evidence to suggest that not all treatments now offered across the spectrum of health services are effective and humane. It is therefore perfectly reasonable for those who hold financial control to request evidence not merely about comparative levels of service, but also about the impact in human terms to be expected from changes in service levels. What they are not entitled to do is to close their eyes to the human effects of their decisions.

5

Conclusions and Implications

The conclusions of the study are linked to its objectives and concern the provision and analysis of data; tentative policy implications; and recommendations for future data collection.

Data Provision and Analysis

The study set out to try to provide reasonably reliable data on health-care expenditures in the ten countries, and to determine the comparability of the totals by analyzing them in four complementary ways. In reviewing the results, it is much easier to point out the gaps than to judge the reliability and comparability of the data. The gaps in the main data tables are relatively few (see the summary in figure 5-1). In table 3-3 the trend information is incomplete, particularly for the early years, but there is nevertheless some indication of historical development in every country included. There is difficulty in table 4-2 in differentiating the ownership and control of institutions and services, between government on the one hand and public non-profit on the other, and between the latter and private, for-profit ownership. This difficulty stems partly from lack of recording in some countries (especially concerning the private sector) and partly from the natural shading of sectors into one another. Although the resource analysis, summarized in table 4-3, and the supporting manpower information in table 4-5, provide enough information to show the broad pattern, there are still many gaps. Recording is relatively complete for public agencies, particularly hospitals. Unfortunately, by itself this has little value. For the private sector the data are incomplete almost everywhere, and even in the public sector community-health programs are far less well documented than hospitals. Census information does not fill the gap, since it tends not to capture data on people who work in health services in a supporting capacity not specific to the health field. Table 4-12, which contains the breakdown by service, is sufficiently complete to reveal major complexities of definition, for example in the classification of physicians' fees for attending patients in the hospital, and of hospital-based ambulatory care. The discrepancies mainly affect the comparability of particular items in table 4-12 rather than the comparability of total expenditure, although there are some difficulties over education, research, and especially the frontier between health-care expenditure and social welfare.

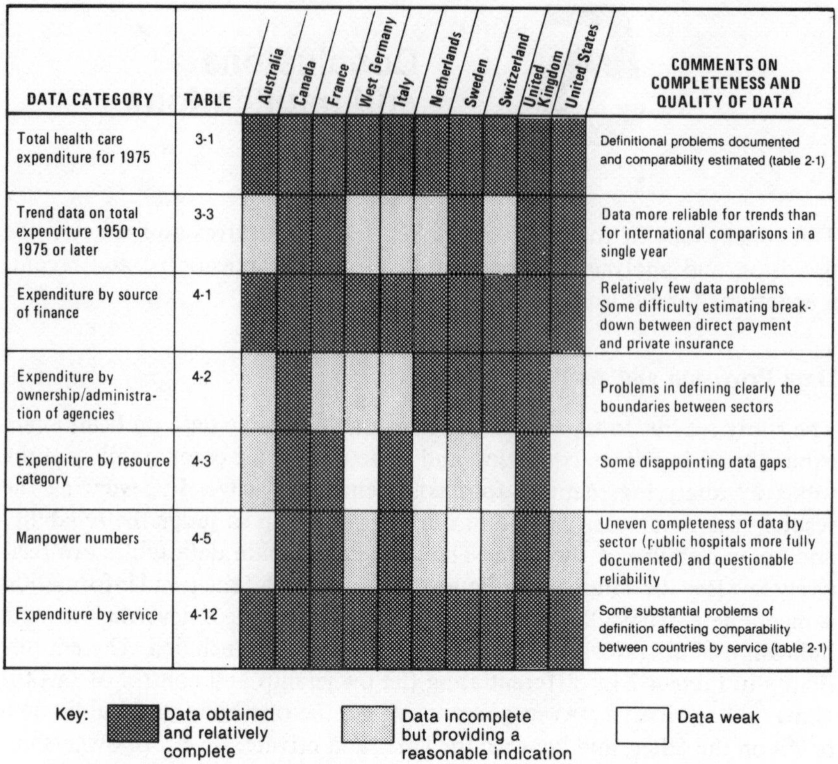

DATA CATEGORY	TABLE	Australia	Canada	France	West Germany	Italy	Netherlands	Sweden	Switzerland	United Kingdom	United States	COMMENTS ON COMPLETENESS AND QUALITY OF DATA
Total health care expenditure for 1975	3-1											Definitional problems documented and comparability estimated (table 2-1)
Trend data on total expenditure 1950 to 1975 or later	3-3											Data more reliable for trends than for international comparisons in a single year
Expenditure by source of finance	4-1											Relatively few data problems Some difficulty estimating break-down between direct payment and private insurance
Expenditure by ownership/administration of agencies	4-2											Problems in defining clearly the boundaries between sectors
Expenditure by resource category	4-3											Some disappointing data gaps
Manpower numbers	4-5											Uneven completeness of data by sector (public hospitals more fully documented) and questionable reliability
Expenditure by service	4-12											Some substantial problems of definition affecting comparability between countries by service (table 2-1)

Key: Data obtained and relatively complete   Data incomplete but providing a reasonable indication   Data weak

Figure 5-1. Summary of Data Obtained and Data Gaps

Concern about the reliability of the data is less justified than concern about comparability. The main guarantee of reliability is the high caliber of the people who helped with the study in each country. All the totals can be documented from an authoritative national statistical source or study, and so in nearly all cases can the analysis by source of finance (table 4-1). Estimates in the other tables do not affect the validity of the totals and are in most cases based on close knowledge of the data sources and the way in which the health system works in the country concerned. Inevitably, there is more solid documentation for some countries, such as the United States, France, and Sweden, than for, say, Italy and Switzerland, where analysis depends on the heroic efforts of a few individuals.

Comparability is a much greater problem because we still lack an internationally agreed set of definitions. There are many instances in which one could with equal justification include or exclude a particular item when constructing a national record of health-care expenditures. For example, it is not obvious one way or the other (in the absence of an agreed set of definitions) whether preclinical medical education, or patients' traveling costs, or day centers for the elderly should be included. Different people quite legitimately take different views, for reasons that seem good to them, and it is very difficult in a retrospective study to make sure that one has checked every component adequately for all the possible differences in definition. In the present study the main items that health-care spending comprises were first defined, so that at least the information was sought to a standard specification in a standard format. The inclusion of a four-faceted breakdown of expenditure (by source of finance; by ownership or administration of the institutions and agencies; by resource category; and by service) also made it more likely that definitional problems would be identified. An analysis of a single facet (such as source of finance or expenditure by service) would almost certainly miss anomalies in other facets. And a list of questions about potential definitional problems was used in collecting and reviewing the data for each country.

Some relatively obvious, but serious, traps were avoided by these means. It is common enough to find, for example, French figures quoted in international studies in the relatively narrow definition of *consommation médicale finale* (excluding research, education, preventive activities, and some aspects of administration) rather than in the broader definition of *dépense nationale de santé*, without adequate consideration of comparability with other figures quoted. Similarly, German figures containing cash benefits are sometimes used, because that is how the figures are usually quoted in Germany. And figures for the United Kingdom often ignore some non-National Health Service spending, such as private-sector spending, and medical services for the armed forces.

Thus, although some traps have been avoided, others undoubtedly remain. Table 2-1 attempts to draw together information on these definitional matters for each country's data and to assess in broad terms how the differences affect comparability. Owing to definitional problems, total health-care expenditure as reported may (in my opinion) be some 5-10 percent low for Switzerland and up to 5 percent low for Australia, Italy, and the Netherlands. When it was possible to adjust the data by adding or subtracting specific identifiable items, this has been done, for example by omitting from the Italian figures bank interest forced on the health system by government policy. When such adjustments could be made only by assuming that what applies in one country must apply in another, it seemed better not to do so. Instead I have tried to point out the differences in coverage and definition, so that people are aware of them and can take them into account.

Although imperfections in the figures undoubtedly remain, they are unlikely to be seriously misleading, partly because an inaccuracy or inconsistency even in several cells of the analysis would be unlikely to make a major difference in the patterns that emerge. The only aspect that is still of serious concern is the frontier with welfare services in the treatment of the handicapped and the elderly. This particular boundary cannot be precise, since the care required so often calls for a range of resources in varying combinations. At times medical and nursing skills are most needed, at other times social work or housing or cash may be more important. Therefore, people should be crossing the frontier all the time; the less rigid it is, the better. Where it is drawn in funding terms is arbitrary, depending usually on whether a particular activity was originally administered by a health agency, such as a hospital, or by a social welfare organization. Since the line is somewhat blurred in each country, it is very difficult indeed to be clear about international comparability. Moreover, it is also hard to distinguish variations in labeling from substantive differences in approach. For example, West Germany, in particular, makes extensive use of spas, which could be excluded from the definition of health care and considered instead as part of the tourist or leisure industry. In my view, however, they can properly be seen as an aspect of health services in Germany that is not precisely matched in most of the other countries. Similarly, the size of the nursing-home sector varies substantially among countries, and yet (unless the name conceals an identity that has nothing to do with nursing) it seems proper to include this sector.

There is no question but that further research will show the present study to have been imperfect. That, however, is the way of all scientific investigation, and leads on to what is said at the end of this chapter about continuing data collection. It is hoped that the basis for the summary figures is sufficiently clearly documented that their publication will itself help to identify any errors and discrepancies that they may contain, and will thus contribute to further development. Meanwhile, I believe there is enough validity in the figures given in chapters 3 and 4 and in the relationships suggested to provide grist for other people's thinking.

Policy Implications

In part this study simply confirms and updates the conclusions of earlier work. For example, it confirms the increase of health-care expenditures of about 1 percent of gross national product in the 1950s [6], and 1.5 percent or more in the 1960s [7], and the clear relationship between national spending and national wealth. The wealthier a country is, the higher tends to be the proportion of its wealth spent on health care [27]. The apparently inexorable rises in costs are attributed to causes similar to those identified by others [21,24,48]. The tendency for government to become increasingly involved in the funding and (to a lesser extent) the administration of services has been noted elsewhere [8]. So has the lack of any clear correspondence between health-care spending and needs [6] or results [28,29] insofar as these can at present be measured. The important caution is added (with which many previous writers would agree) that it would be unwise to assume from this lack of correspondence that health-care expenditures make no difference. On the contrary, spending levels can strongly influence the levels of ascertainment of need and of service provision; although there is no guarantee that high spending will by itself achieve high value, and our measures of the impact of services are totally inadequate.

The main change from the findings of previous studies is a recent interruption, and in some cases a reversal, of trends that had become the accepted pattern in the 1950s and 1960s. The evidence is far from complete, and the effect varies markedly from country to country, but the signs are there. For example, whereas the average increase in health-care spending in these countries in the first half of the 1970s approached 1.5 percent of GNP (almost as much as in the whole of the 1960s), since then the increase relative to GNP has halted, except in Sweden, Australia, and the United States (see table 5-1 and table 3-3). Another change in trend (for example, in Australia) is a reduction in the proportion of health-care expenditures financed by government.

By the early 1970s it was clear that a crisis would soon arise in health-care spending [29]. For at least twenty years, throughout the developed world, annual increases in health-care expenditures had consistently outstripped increases in national income. The factors that had fueled this increase had not spent their force, and one could safely predict that health-care expenditures would not quickly reach a natural plateau, either in money

Table 5-1
Changes in National Health-Care Spending as a Percentage of GNP

Country	1950-1955	1955-1960	1960-1965	1965-1970	1970-1975	1975-1977
Australia	—	—	+0.2	+0.3	+1.5	+0.9
Canada	+0.3	+1.3	+0.5	+1.0	+0.0	+0.0
France	+1.1	+0.2	+1.1	+0.6	+1.5	+0.0
West Germany	—	—	—	—	+3.0	-0.2
Italy	—	—	—	(+1.0)	(+1.1)	-0.7
Netherlands	—	+0.5	+0.8	+1.0	+1.8	+0.1
Sweden	+0.7	+0.6	+0.9	+1.8	+1.1	+1.3
Switzerland	—	—	—	—	—	+0.0
United Kingdom	-0.5	+0.4	+0.1	+0.4	+1.2	-0.3
United States	-0.1	+0.9	+0.9	+1.4	+1.0	+0.4
	1.5 (÷5)	3.9 (÷6)	.4.5 (÷7)	7.5 (÷8)	12.2 (÷9)	1.5 (÷10)
Average	+0.3	+0.65	+0.64	+0.94	+1.36	+0.15

Source: Table 3-3.

terms or as a percentage of GNP. On the other hand, governments, which had been the principal paymasters for increased health-care spending, would be more sensitive to further increases now that health care had become a very substantial component of public expenditure. The clash was bound to come eventually. It came earlier than it would otherwise have done because of the worsening macroeconomic position facing governments in the developed world in the 1970s, particularly after the oil crisis of late 1973. Moreover, the sharp reduction in economic growth coincided in many of the Western developed countries with a widespread disillusionment with government in general and with welfare programs in particular.

At this point it is worth reconsidering Seale's general theory of national expenditure on health care [23]. Formulated before the large increases in spending in the late 1950s and the 1960s, the theory was as follows: The proportion of the GNP of a nation devoted to medical care tends to remain constant. It rises during national economic depressions and it falls during wars. A persistent rise in real per-capita GNP will tend to result in a very gradual increase in the proportion.

In light of more recent developments, the theory should perhaps be replaced by one along the following lines: Health-care spending is very closely related to the means available. The higher a nation's GNP, the higher tends to be the proportion of that GNP related to health care. The proportion will tend to rise everywhere in periods of sustained prosperity. In periods of economic difficulty the pattern will be more diverse. Because of the strong pressures for continuing expansion within the health-care system, national expenditure will continue to rise in countries where the controls over health-care expenditures are weak or fragmented. National expenditure may well fall relative to GNP where controls are tight, depending on other perceived priorities. Ultimately, the amount spent, the way it is spent, and the value received for it, depend on choices about behavior and the use of resources at many levels in the health-care system and in society as a whole.

The climate for health services has thus changed radically in the last decade. No government would now subscribe to the view expressed by a politician in the 1960s that "Health care shall cost what it has to cost. We will pay" [49]. Although the timing and severity of the onset of the colder climate has varied, it has arrived in all these countries; the governments concerned have applied the financial brakes and tightened their control over public expenditures on health care.

In most cases the initial moves were directed at prices, including a tougher attitude toward the negotiation of physicians' fee levels and hospital per-diem rates, and a strong wish to set these rates in advance. Since price control leaves the quantity and mix of services unaffected, governments also quickly showed interest in measures designed to limit total expenditure, for example by switching hospitals to global budgets (unaffected by service levels during the year in question); by changing the basis of physicians' remuneration wherever possible (to a salary basis in Swedish outpatient departments, to a capitation basis in some American health-maintenance organizations); and by altering the open-ended commitment by one level of government to another (as in Canada) or by the social-insurance funds to the health system (as in Italy).

Wherever effective systems of budgetary control existed, the limits were tightened and allowances for discretionary development of services were reduced or eliminated. Conventional budgetary systems tended to become less effective as inflation rates rose. The response (at least in Canada and the United Kingdom) was the imposition of cash limits, fixed at a level that did not necessarily fully reflect inflation. Budgetary controls have proved tightest where they rested in few hands and looser where they were fragmented, as in Sweden and the United States.

That such financial measures had an effect is undoubted (see figure 3-12 and table 3-3 for varying periods from 1972 onward for Canada, France, West Germany, Italy, Sweden, the United Kingdom, and the United States). But their main impact was likely to be temporary, since they would not affect most of the causes, discussed in chapter 3, underlying the historical increase in health-care spending. For longer-term control, financial measures would not by themselves be sufficient. If governments wanted to achieve long-term control, limits would also have to be placed on the real resource inputs that determine expenditures in the long run.

All the governments covered by this survey show growing awareness of this fact, and some have demonstrated a ready aptitude to learn quickly how to control these real resource inputs. Where attention should be concentrated is apparent from the resource facet of the analysis in chapter 4 and can be summarized diagrammatically (figure 5-2). Thus personnel numbers and wage rates matter most, followed by various equipment and supply items, particularly drugs. A 5 percent change in personnel costs changes total health-care costs by 3 percent ($5/100 \times 60/100$); a similar change in prescribed drug costs has an impact of 0.5 percent ($5/100 \times 10/100$). Around the outside of the diagram are stated, in crude terms, how that particular element of costs can be influenced, for example by limiting numbers or wage rates, or by substituting lower-cost for higher-cost personnel. Two points are more important than appears on the face of the diagram. The first, discussed more fully in chapter 3, is the crucial position of doctors as prescribers of services. The impact of their number and prescribing behavior is far greater than their, say, 17 percent of direct costs indicates; and they are crucial to the management of all health-care resources [50]. A second influential determinant is the size and scope of the hospital system. While the number of hospital beds (table 4-14) is a very

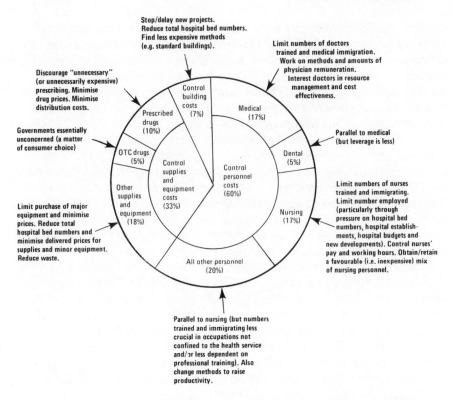

Figure 5-2. Resource Control—An Effective but Limited Approach

imprecise comparative measure, since it says nothing about the range and intensity of work done, there remains substantial truth in Roemer's Law that all available beds will be filled [51]. As we have seen (table 4-11), hospitals account for a substantial portion of total health-care spending, while treating a relatively small proportion of the total episodes of illness (figure 4-11). This is perfectly sensible, granted the heterogeneity of health-care needs, from the simple and relatively minor to the very serious and complex. Nevertheless, from a resource-control viewpoint it is logical enough to concentrate attention on the hospital sector, including bed numbers in the system as a whole; senior medical staffing and admitting privileges; staff numbers and grades: and major equipment. As Mr. Saul Miller, Health Minister of Manitoba, succinctly expressed it, this reflects government acceptance of the Willy Sutton principle. Willy Sutton was once asked why, as an expert thief, he concentrated his attention on banks. "Because", he replied, "that's where the money is".

Besides concern with resource control in the system, there is also the possibility of reversing the historical trend (illustrated, for example, in figure 4-2) toward reliance on public-sector financing. Right-wing governments, in particular, have been attracted by the idea of some shift back to consumer payment, through direct charges at the time of use (as in France, and for dental and optical services and prescribed drugs in the United Kingdom) and through private-sector insurance (as in Australia).

Once they have introduced measures to control public-sector costs, ministries of finance may well turn with relief from health services to other problems. But these steps are negative, whereas for anyone genuinely concerned about health standards and the well-being of the sick and handicapped, financial control must *always* be secondary. Financial control is a necessary discipline and constraint, but the most disciplined and leanest health system in the world would be a bad system if it led to low standards of care and poor results relative to what the country concerned could reasonably afford.

The challenge is not merely to limit, but also to choose in an informed way where to set the limits, and to obtain the best results one can within those limits. This is well expressed in the concept of the "medical commons" [25]: a finite space within which resources are used more or less effectively and equitably to meet the health-care needs of a whole society. It is not just a matter of limiting physician numbers through barriers to immigration and medical-school expansion, but of assessing thoughtfully what numbers and mix of skills, across the whole range of health-related occupations, will produce the best overall results at a tolerable price, and of trying to take the steps to develop and deploy them. Similarly, it is not merely a question of recognizing the truth of Roemer's Law that any hospital bed is likely to be filled, and of therefore paring down bed numbers, but also of seeking the range and balance of preventive, curing, and caring services that will together do the most that is possible, within each community's means, to avoid and relieve human suffering and handicap. Since the medical commons are themselves only part of society's total resources, there is always the question of where the boundary should be set in order to take account of other needs and desires. These are as tough and important problems as mankind faces in any field. There is no perfect or permanent answer to them, not only because of their complexity, but also because human knowledge and skills develop, and the resources available change.

It is inescapable, for the reasons given in chapter 3, that societies find ways of responding on a communal basis, whatever the part played by the private sector. While it is by no means essential that government try to handle all these problems by itself, it is inescapable that society, and therefore government, be concerned about the working of the whole. For these problems to be tackled positively, rather than with the aim of simply minimizing public expenditure, would call for competence far greater than that which any country can yet display. Knowledge is required across the full range of services, geographic areas, and client groups and conditions, as to the relative effectiveness and costs of different methods and resource-distribution patterns. When there is a strong case for change in approach or balance (as there may well be in, for example, strengthening primary care and improving the care of the mentally ill and handicapped, the elderly, and people living in deprived communities), the skills to bring this about are formidable. Where governments have moved into this field at all, they have underestimated the leadership, trust, and patience required to alter health services materially without doing more harm than good. It is far easier to destroy something in health-care delivery than it is to create something better. Most of the time it is best to proceed by encouraging and learning from new initiatives that seem good, while keeping the rest of the operation running as smoothly as possible.

In the mid- and late 1970s the spotlight has been on health-care expenditures. Financial control has received attention almost to the exclusion of everything else. But since countries that did not already have effective controls have acted or will act to put them in place, this will soon be yesterday's problem. Today's problem can be expressed more positively as that of pursuing value for money in health services—a more exciting and more formidable task than mere financial control, necessary as that is.

Even when countries develop greater skill in managing their health systems, there is a constant danger of their being too supply-side (and service-provision) oriented. For there is an important sense in which the politician who said, "Health care shall cost what it has to cost," was wiser in his naiveté than the more sober governments of today. As one supports and guides the enormous complex represented by health services, one should always also be concerned with doing something useful about any problem of handicap, suffering, or distress. If resource constraints, access difficulties, or even lack of present knowledge make it hard to help someone who needs help, one cannot rest satisfied. A way must be found to work within the constraint or to remove it. Of course, what can usefully be done will not always lie within the ambit of health services. Road accidents, alcoholism, and lung cancer are much better prevented, by whatever means, than patched up after the event. This in no way lessens the obligation to seek a way to help. And even at the aggregate levels of national statistics like age-specific mortality ratios, it looks as though there are important variations in these problems. In Sweden, for example, despite its excellent overall statistics, there are major mortality losses from age 15 onward through accidents (principally not automobile accidents), injury, suicide, and psychiatric disorders. In the United Kingdom these problems are far less frequent, whereas from age 35 onward circulatory disease, lung cancer, and respiratory disease are much graver hazards than in Sweden. The U.S. and Canadian patterns fall between those of the United Kingdom and Sweden, with some of the worse characteristics of both and (at least up to 1974) worse automobile-accident figures than either. Although many of these problems fall outside the health-care field as traditionally defined, they do not fall outside the field of health policy.

Just as these variations exist at the national level and suggest some of the points where there may be room for improvement, so also there is value in defining local health problems and failures to meet needs adequately. The argument that it is better not to look for problems when resources are already stretched is an unworthy one. Apart from humane concern (since there is absolutely no guarantee that the unseen need is unimportant in terms of human suffering), a defined, serious, remediable problem provides the best stimulus for change in the health system. The principal challenge in health care has always been and will always be how to minimize human suffering and handicap. Recognizing this is made more urgent by the increased (and necessary) skills developed in public financial control. When there is weak control over money, someone, somewhere can be counted on to find the means to tackle a neglected problem. When the control limits are tight, this is no longer true. Thus constructive dissatisfaction with things as they are, and with neglected needs and low standards, becomes absolutely vital.

Conversely, established practices and trends must be questioned. Technical interventions are by no means always justified, particularly when they undermine independence and dignity. The hospice movement [52] is an encouraging example of intelligent and compassionate concern for those who face pain and likely death. It is not an antitechnological approach, for it makes extensive use of drugs and other weapons in the medical armory; but it subordinates the use of technology to concern for the individual and awareness of the inevitability of death.

More broadly, medical services must not become a substitute for self-help, improved community networks of social support, and a realistic acceptance of the human condition [53]. Faced with resource limits and the virtually limitless potential for human "dis-ease," overreliance on medical services would be madness. But it is equally important to remember how powerful are the capabilities of modern health services to relieve pain, assist the disabled to live a fuller life, and comfort and care for the sick. Access to these capabilities should not depend on wealth or privilege, but on need and fairness within the limits that society can afford.

The appropriate model for health-care management in the 1980s is much less simple than cost containment, and more exciting. Again, in a very crude way, it can be summarized diagrammatically (see figure 5-3).

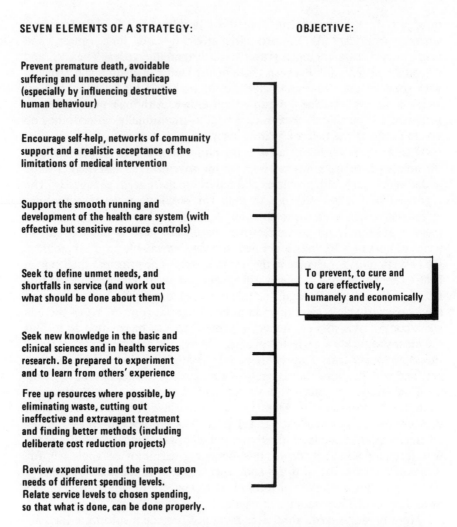

SEVEN ELEMENTS OF A STRATEGY:

OBJECTIVE:

Prevent premature death, avoidable
suffering and unnecessary handicap
(especially by influencing destructive
human behaviour)

Encourage self-help, networks of community
support and a realistic acceptance of the
limitations of medical intervention

Support the smooth running and
development of the health care system (with
effective but sensitive resource controls)

Seek to define unmet needs, and
shortfalls in service (and work out
what should be done about them)

To prevent, to cure and
to care effectively,
humanely and economically

Seek new knowledge in the basic and
clinical sciences and in health services
research. Be prepared to experiment
and to learn from others' experience

Free up resources where possible, by
eliminating waste, cutting out
ineffective and extravagant treatment
and finding better methods (including
deliberate cost reduction projects)

Review expenditure and the impact upon
needs of different spending levels.
Relate service levels to chosen spending,
so that what is done, can be done properly.

Figure 5-3. A Crude Strategic Concept for Health Care in the 1980s

Influencing destructive behavior gives us scope for prevention of unnecessary suffering and handicap and of premature death. Some of the
things that should be done are obvious enough, if the political will exists,
for example enforcement of laws against driving after drinking. There is
also good evidence for others, such as better diet, regular exercise, and no
smoking; reduction of violence and of accidents in the home; avoidance of
environmental hazards; and improved coverage of prenatal care and immunization programs. It would be foolish to pretend that widespread changes

in individual behavior along these lines are easy to achieve, but it is equally true that nobody can yet claim that the effort invested in achieving them compares with the human ingenuity devoted to much more trivial ends.

The next five elements in the diagram are almost self-explanatory against the background of this chapter. Self-help, community networks of support, and a realization of the limitations of medical intervention are all essential to the responsible use of health-care resources. Equally, existing institutions, agencies, and services require support and guidance. Whatever their imperfections, they have developed organically in response to perceived need, are trying to do a conscientious job, and in most instances carry a big workload. Sometimes revolutionary change may be justified, but it always exacts a high price in terms of dislocation and disorientation. Short of revolutionary change, evolutionary development happens continuously in any lively service and can be nudged in what seems the right direction. When it does not happen, but appears to be required, one must try to find an opportunity for new stimulus to arise from the recognition of a major unmet need or deficiency in service. I feel it is a fundamental error to insulate people from new stimuli through distrust of their responses. This appears too often to be what provincial and state governments have done in Canada and Australia, by debarring many hospital boards from undertaking community programs. Meanwhile, the effectiveness of present and proposed treatment methods should be constantly questioned in order to learn how they can be improved. And expenditure of all kinds should be reviewed analytically in a search for acceptable ways to reduce costs.

The final heading in the diagram needs a little more explanation. For the future it is inevitable that countries will set health-care-expenditure limits (at least for public-sector spending) more firmly than in the past. And the limits may well be tighter than anyone would wish, depending on the means available and on other priorities. It is up to those concerned with health policy to see that expenditure is not discussed without also discussing, in a realistic way, what the money will buy. Too often governments have taken the line that health services expenditure will be cut but there must be no reduction in services to patients. This stance is dishonest. Funding and service levels are interdependent. At any specified funding level there are some things that should be done and others that should not. In the long run, to promise a level of service that is beyond one's means to give is bound to lead to deteriorating standards and to frustration. It is far more honest, and ultimately more sensible, to consider funding and service levels simultaneously and, if necessary, face up to restrictions of some services.

Looking ahead into the 1980s, it is clear that the problems recently encountered in health-care finance and policy will not go away. A sudden resumption of untroubled economic growth is improbable and would not in any case provide a complete or lasting solution. Health services can readily absorb the increases in financial and other resources available to them—and still have an appetite for more. Governments having become heavily committed to the health-care sector, they now have few strategic options; and each of these has its dangers.

One option, in theory at least, is to elect to let past trends continue; but governments that take this route will face continuing sharp increases in health-care expenditures. An alternative is to withdraw as much as possible from the responsibility for ensuring access to health care and to try strictly to limit government's financial exposure. The danger here is that variations in access to care and in the quality of care will markedly increase, depending on the capacity of individuals and local communities to pay. Such variations may be tolerable for consumer goods, but are they tolerable for health care? A third option is to choose certain limited objectives for government involvement, such as the protection of public health and the provision of a "safety net" for the poor and catastrophically sick, and to decline to take any responsibility for the working of the rest of the health-care system. The problem with this approach is that expenditures will still continue to rise dramatically in the health-care sector as a whole, since the public sector cannot be insulated from the rest, and that government-provided services will look increasingly threadbare compared with private ones.

In my opinion none of these options is sustainable for long. Governments will not be able to ignore continuing uncontrolled increases in publicly financed health-care expenditures, nor will these expenditures stabilize of their own accord. On the other hand, the hardships for the least fortunate and the resentments that would result from the second option would soon force government into a stance of at least limited involvement and responsibility. While it is much more defensible to select limited fields for government intervention, one cannot ignore some of the broader problems of the health sector, nor the interrelationships and comparisons between government and other programs.

There are of course a variety of options remaining, from that of a national-health service to a situation in which government itself runs few health services but regulates, influences, and helps to finance a multiplicity of health agencies. In political terms there are enormous differences between these options. In either case, however, many of the same problems arise and many of the same skills are required. Thus, the broad strategy proposed in figure 5-3 is relevant to both. What ultimately matters is how effectively and humanely, within its resources, any society responds to the wide variety of human needs, including the needs of people who have neither wealth, position, nor political influence, nor even a condition of compelling scientific interest.

The 1980s seems likely to be a decade of uncertainty and divergent trends and policies in the health-care sector as governments react in different ways to the problems highlighted in this study. Whereas in retrospect the main trends of the 1950s and 1960s were common, resulting in steadily rising health-care expenditures and ever-increasing government involvement, the trends in the 1980s are likely to be hesitant and divergent. Some governments will ignore the problem for as long as possible. Others will take a firm and hard line to reduce their exposure to rising costs, whatever the impact may be in terms of growing differences in health-care standards for the rich and the poor. Others will concentrate their attention on controlling inputs and prices across the whole range of public and private services. But in the long term the most important questions of health policy are too complex for any of these approaches to be an adequate total response. And any modern society should be judged by, among other measures, how its sick and handicapped are cared for and assisted. That is an issue of public policy that no one can ultimately escape. It calls for, among other qualities, sensitivity and generosity.

Continuing Data Collection

If financial control is yesterday's problem, why bother about collecting information on expenditures and trying to improve its promptness, comprehensiveness, and quality? It is perfectly true that many of the most important things to know, such as the nature of needs that are unmet and of standards that should be improved, will require special studies and will not be reported, given the current state of knowledge, within any likely routine system of international data collection on health expenditures. Nevertheless, I believe it is ludicrous to neglect information on what is spent now and on the key expenditure components and trends. Since there are no absolute standards in health care, one can safely ignore neither present resource limits and uses nor the insights given and the questions raised by comparison. Although there will have to be detailed studies to pin down the reasons for variations in expenditure patterns and the conclusions to be drawn from them, there is also a need to see the detail within a broad analytic context. This helps to show what is important financially and why, and to give an insight into the nature of health-care sytems and the financial characteristics of health services in particular countries.

The time is overdue for international agreement on data collection about health expenditures. It is foolish to continue to rely on the initiative of individuals, whose immediate difficulty is that, because there is no agreement on even the most basic analytic framework and definitions, the task is bound to be time consuming and the results patchy. Brian Abel-Smith's study [6] took ten years, and the present study has taken three. With an agreed chart of accounts, a mechanism for international collaboration, and appropriate data collection and analysis within countries, the information could be provided much more promptly and reliably. This should certainly be done, but there is still room for debate on the best method of doing it.

Based on the experience of the present study, and without wishing to preempt the discussion, I suggest six steps:

1. An international body such as the World Health Organization should act as convenor and enabler so that experts draw up an agreed chart of accounts as soon as possible and establish an international mechanism for regular data submission and publication.

2. The chart of accounts should be multifaceted. The initial hypothesis that a four-faceted analysis was more valuable than any single facet has, in my opinion, been substantiated in this book. The method has some of the inherent internal checks of double-entry bookkeeping and is more illuminating than, say, an analysis of sources of health-care funding on its own.

3. Among many matters of definition that the international group must decide and record unambiguously, some of the most important are the boundary between health-care spending and social welfare (especially in services for the elderly and handicapped); the classification of physicians' fees and hospital-based ambulatory care in relation to hospital costs; and the yardstick to be used for national income (GNP or gross domestic product, at market or factor prices, for single years or on a trend basis).

4. It is urgently necessary for most countries to improve their information on the resource facet of the analysis, including manpower. As tables 4-3 and 4-5 and figure 5-1 show, there are at present major gaps, particularly because data-collection systems concentrate on public-sector institutions, frequently leaving out community services and the private sector; yet manpower and other key resource information cannot be compared across countries without combining the two, because the mix between private and public varies so markedly among countries.

5. Consideration should also be given to adding (initially or later) a fifth facet of expenditure by category of persons served and their characteristics, including age and type of disease or handicap. No routine analysis will cover needs and benefits adequately, but this fifth facet would at least provide the right context in which to ask questions about them. Initially one could concentrate on the elderly and the very young, since it is for these age groups that needs are greatest and expenditures highest.

6. It is essential to have in each country a group of people committed to the continuing collection and analysis of national health-care-expenditure data, linked to the international network already proposed. Such a group can be outside government (like CREDOC in Paris or the Istituto per la

ricerca di Economia Sanitaria in Milan) or inside it (like the Department of Health and Human Services, in Washington; Health and Welfare Canada in Ottawa; and, most recently, the Commonwealth Department of Health in Canberra). Either way, the existence of such committed units, and the development of international links among them, are essential to further progress in this field.

Appendix A: Health-Expenditure Analysis: Standard Chart of Accounts Used in the Study

	1974	1975	Notes
Basic data			

1. Population (thousands)

2. GNP

3. GNP per capita

Health expenditure by source of finance[a]

4. Public
   (a) General taxation
   (b) Compulsory insurance/social security
   (c) Other (specify)

5. Consumers
   (a) Voluntary insurance
   (b) Direct payment
   (c) Other (specify)

6. Other (specify)

7. Total expenditure
   (a) Total
   (b) Per capita
   (c) Percentage of GNP
   (d) Percentage of GDP

Health expenditure by ownership/administration of channel of provision[a]

8. Government institutions (state-owned and -run)

9. Nongovernment, not for profit

10. Private, for-profit institutions and contractors

11. Other (specify)

12. Total (8-11)

Appendix A *(continued)*

	1974	1975	Notes

Health expenditure by service

13. Hospitals (current, excluding
    amortization)
    (a) Inpatient
    (b) Outpatient

14. Hospitals (capital)

15. Care outside hospitals
    (a) Primary care
    (b) Specialist care
    (c) Capital expenditure

16. Self-care

17. Other services
    (a) Public health
    (b) Research
    (c) Education
    (d) Other

18. Administration

19. Other

20. Total

	Cost	Number	Cost	Number

Health expenditure by resource

Manpower

21. Doctors
    (a) General practice
    (b) All other

    Dentists
    (a) General Practice
    (b) All other

22. Nurses (qualified)

23. Nurses (other)

    Total nursing

24. Professional and technical

25. Administrative and clerical and
    auxiliary

26. Total manpower

Appendix A *(continued)*

	1974	*1975*	*Notes*
27. Pharmaceuticals a. Prescribed b. OTC drugs			
28. Equipment and supplies			
29. Buildings			
Other			
Total			

Note: It may be possible to present the data in these sections by a matrix of which one side represents the source of finance and the other the channel of provision.

Appendix B:
Checklist for Definition
of Expenditure on
Health Services

1. *Coverage*: Does the estimate include the cost of health services provided for the armed forces (1) at home, (2) abroad? Are there any separate health services—for such groups as the police, residents of prisons, transport workers, and industrial workers at factories—which are excluded?
2. On what basis is a separation made between hospital services and social-welfare institutions for (1) the aged, (2) the mentally retarded, (3) alcoholics, (4) drug addicts, (5) cripples, (6) convalescents, (7) ex-mental patients? Is the distinction based on the name of the institution, whether it is run by a doctor, whether it employs trained nurses, or other criteria?
3. What travel costs of patients are included: (1) travel by ambulance; (2) private travel by taxi, public transport, or private car to visit (a) a hospital, (b) a doctor, (c) a dentist, (d) a pharmacist?
4. Is all cost of education and training for (1) doctors, (2) dentists, (3) nurses, (4) pharmacists, (5) medical auxiliaries included, or on what principle is a division made?
5. Does it include the cost of (1) education for children who are hospital patients, (2) education for the mentally retarded in or out of the hospital, (3) religious services for hospital patients, (4) social-work services to sick persons *in* or *out* of the hospital, (5) cash allowances given to long-term and poor hospital residents, (6) domestic-help services provided to sick persons?
6. What environmental services are included? Does it include only the costs of medical supervision of (1) shops, offices, and restaurants; (2) water supply; (3) refuse collection; (4) sewage disposal; (5) air-pollution control? Or does it include the *provision* of (1) water, (2) sewage disposal, (3) public toilet facilities, (4) disinfection, (5) burial of poor persons, (6) forensic medical services?
7. What costs of medical research are included—only for research undertaken in hospitals or for all medical research?
8. What capital construction costs are included: (1) hospital, (2) ambulatory clinics—preventative and curative; (3) the offices of private doctors, dentists, and other professional personnel; (4) the construction of factories to manufacture pharmaceuticals or other health-care supplies?

9. Does the running cost include an element for the depreciation of hospitals and other health-care buildings, and on what principle is the element for depreciation calculated, for example historical cost or replacement cost based on what depreciation period?

10. Is the estimate based on expenditure of patients or insurers (social security or voluntary) or on the cost of providing the service? This problem arises particularly with hospitals, which may accumulate deficits if their revenues do not cover their running costs.

11. What administrative costs are included, for example, (1) the ministry of health or other ministries responsible for health services or social-security health services; (2) the costs of social-security agencies and insurers in collecting subscriptions and paying benefits?

12. Are charitable services provided by members of religious orders counted at cost or at the market price of purchasing such services on the market from persons not members of religious orders?

Appendix C:
National Data
Summaries for the Ten
Countries Included in
the Survey

Table C-1
Australia
(millions of Australian dollars, unless stated otherwise)

	1974-1975	1974-1975 Percentage	1975-1976	1975-1976 Percentage	Notes (1)
Basic data					
1. Population (thousands)	13,420		13,709		(2)
2. GNP	NA		NA		
GDP	60,149		70,825		(3)
3. GNP per capita	NA		NA		
GDP per capita (dollars)	4,482		5,166		
Health expenditure by source of finance					
4. Public					
(a) General taxation	2,640	62.7	3,980	73.5	
(b) Public insurance	70	1.7	90	1.7	
	2,710	64.4	4,070	75.2	
5. Consumers					(4)
(a) Private insurance	580	13.8	430	7.9	
(b) Direct payment	891	21.1	860	15.9	
	1,471	34.9	1,290	23.8	
6. Other	29	0.7	50	1.0	
7. Total expenditure					
(a) Total	4,210	100.0	5,410	100.0	(5)
(b) Per capita (dollars)	314		395		
(c) Percentage of GNP	—		—		
(d) Percentage of GDP	7.0		7.6		
Health expenditure by ownership/administration of channel of provision					
8. Government institutions (state-owned and -run)	2,271	53.9	2,944	54.4	
9. Nongovernment, not for profit					
	1,939	46.1	2,466	45.6	(6)
10. Private, for-profit institutions and contractors					
11. Other	—		—		
12. Total (8-11)	4,210	100.0	5,410	100.0	
Health expenditure by service					
13. Hospitals (current)					
(a) Inpatient	1,834	43.6	2,355	43.5	
(b) Outpatient	310	7.4	400	7.4	
	2,144	51.0	2,755	50.9	
14. Hospitals (capital)	250	5.9	320	5.9	
	2,394	56.9	3,075	56.8	(7)
15. Care outside hospitals					
(a) Primary care	1,264	30.0	1,676	31.0	
(b) Specialist care					
(c) Capital expenditure	45	1.1	60	1.1	
16. Self-medication	208	4.9	228	4.2	

Table C-1 *(continued)*

	1974-1975	1974-1975 Percentage	1975-1976	1975-1976 Percentage	Notes (1)
17. Other services					
(a) Public health	130	3.1	142	2.6	
(b) Research	19	0.5	24	0.5	
(c) Education	60	1.4	77	1.4	
18. Administration	90	2.1	128	2.4	(7)
19. Other					
20. Total (13-19)	4,210	100.0	5,410	100.0	

	Cost	Percentage	Number	Cost	Percentage	Number
Health expenditure by resource						
Manpower						
21. Doctors						
(a) General practice	(530)	(12.6)	(8,000)	(700)	(12.9)	8,500
(b) All other			(12,400)			13,400
			(20,400)			21,900
Dentists			(4,030)			(4,100)
22. Nurses (qualified)						(49,000)
23. Nurses (other) Total nursing						(8)
24. Professional and technical						
25. Administrative and clerical and auxiliary						
26. Total manpower	2,660	63.2		3,534	65.3	
27. Pharmaceuticals						
(a) Prescribed	354	8.4		388	7.2	
(b) OTC drugs	208	4.9		228	4.2	(9)
	562	13.3		616	11.4	
28. Equipment and supplies	693	16.5		880	16.3	(10)
29. Buildings	295	7.0		380	7.0	(11)
30. Other	—			—		
31. Total (21-30)	4,210	100.0		5,410	100.0	

Sources: The Australian figures were estimated with the help of Dr. J.S. Deeble of the Health Research Project at the Australian National University, Canberra. I am very grateful to him. The principal source is J.S. Deeble, *Health Expenditure in Australia 1960-61 to 1975-76* (Canberra, ANC, 1978). References are to the numbers in the right hand column of the Australian tables.

NA = not available.

Reference notes:

(1) *Dates*: The figures are for fiscal years, which in Australia end on 30 June of the calendar year.

(2) *Population*: These are estimated 31 December totals (the middle of the fiscal year) derived by averaging the preceding and succeeding 30 June totals given in the *Pocket Compendium of Australian Statistics, 1978* (hereafter referred to as the *Compendium*).

(3) *GNP/GDP*: GDP is from the *Compendium*. GNP is not available for Australia from government statistics but would not be substantially different from GDP. (For example, a calendar-1975 GDP estimate derived from these figures and converted to U.S. dollars differs little from the GNP estimate given in the 1978 *World Bank Atlas*.)

Table C-1 *(continued)*

(4) *Expenditure by source of finance*: The breakdown is not available in this form in Deeble's book but was supplied by him. The general-tax funding was overwhelmingly federal in origin, although partly channeled through state and local budgets for spending purposes. Public insurance comprised workers' compensation and automobile insurance. Private insurance (line 5a) represented subscription income for the year. Direct payment was estimated residually from the other figures.

On 1 July 1975 the Whitlam government introduced Medibank. A 28 percent increase in total spending (in money, not real terms) followed in fiscal 1975-1976, as well as a 49 percent increase in estimated total payments for private medical services. Most of the increase was funded by the federal government from general tax revenue, and the general-tax proportion of total health funding (line 4a) rose above 73 percent in that year before dropping back with the subsequent change of government and alterations to the Medibank scheme.

(5) *Total Expenditure*: Inclusions and exclusions are discussed in Deeble, *Health Expenditure*, pp. 9-14 and appendix A. The Australian definition includes all medical services, clinical education (but not the first preclinical year for medical students), research (except when recovered through the price of drugs), and administration of government health departments and of the health-insurance funds. Public-health activities are included, along with the medical supervision of environmental services like water supply and sanitation, but not the services themselves. With respect to the boundary between health and welfare, the main criterion applied was "evidence of curative or palliative intent." On this basis Deeble has tried to exclude the care of the mentally handicapped not suffering from an identifiable illness, and the institutional care of the elderly not undergoing medical treatment. This is a narrower definition than that used in most of the other countries and may result in a somewhat lower estimate of total health-care expenditure. In practice, as elsewhere, one must accept that the boundary between health and welfare is not a precise one and often depends more on the designation of the administering agency than on the substance of the program. All privately arranged transport is excluded, as is some capital expenditure by the private sector. See also table 2-1 for a summary of Australian definitions compared with those for other countries included in the present survey.

(6) *Ownership/administration*: The breakdown is derived from Deeble, *Health Expenditure*, table 1. The allocation between government and nongovernment for 1974-1975 is estimated as follows:

Government	Millions of Australian Dollars	Nongovernment	Millions of Australian Dollars
Commonwealth institutions	137	Private hospitals and nursing homes	391
State hospitals and nursing homes	1,616	Medical services	570
Other medical care (public)	64	Dental and related services	205
Public-health services	130	Drugs	562
Teaching and research	79	Appliances	71
Administrative costs (half of total administrative costs)	45	Administrative costs (half of total administrative costs)	45
	2,071		1,844
Capital	200	Capital	95
	2,271		1,939

For 1975-1976 the allocation was done in exactly the same way. Within the nongovernment sector no breakdown is available between nonprofit and for-profit. By analogy with other countries the following can be classified with reasonable certainty as for-profit:

	Millions of Australian Dollars
Medical services provided by private practitioners and businesses	570
Dental services provided by private practitioners and businesses	205
Drugs	562
Appliances	71
	1,408

The minimum for-profit sector is thus $1,408 million (Australian dollars), or 33.5 percent of total health-care expenditure. Other costs for private hospitals and nursing homes, administration, and capital expenditure, totaling $531 million (12.6 percent of all health-care expenditure) may be either for-profit or nonprofit. Thus, the for-profit sector must fall in the range 33.5-46.1 percent of total health-care costs.

Table C-1 *(continued)*

(7) *Health expenditure by service*: The breakdown is based on Deeble, *Health Expenditure*, table 1. The split between hospital-inpatient and hospital-outpatient costs is not given in that table and is very rough. *Hospital costs as recorded do not include fees charged by private physicians for hospital care.* These would add several percentage points (perhaps 2.5 percent of total expenditure) to hospital costs versus care outside hospitals, but unfortunately no accurate figures are available. Total health-care expenditure would not be affected by the transfer.

(8) *Manpower numbers and costs*: The number of physicians (general practitioners [GPs] and specialists) given for 1975-1976 is the February 1977 figure given in J.C.H. Dewdney, *Australian Health Care Data-Book, 1977* (Sydney, University of New South Wales, 1977), p. 44. The 1974-1975 total for physicians is from Deeble, and the GP-specialist breakdown is estimated from the 1975-1976 proportions. Total physician remuneration is estimated from Dewdney and Deeble at $26,000 per annum for 1974-1975. This is approximately the *net*-earnings figure for tax purposes, after deducting expenses, of doctors in private practice, who constitute a majority of the total. It may well be too high for salaried physicians, but on the other hand it may well understate private-practice earnings. (In calculating total health expenditures, however, the *gross*-earnings figure has been used.)

Numbers of nurses derive from the National Survey of Nursing Personnel at 31 March 1978. An allowance has been made for part-time workers, to reduce the total to an estimated whole-time equivalent.

As in most other countries, there is a dearth of reliable health-manpower statistics, particularly outside the public hospitals. The total is very rough and is based on an estimate from Deeble. Total manpower costs are a residual, arrived at by deducting lines 27-29 from total expenditure.

(9) *Pharmaceuticals*: See Deeble, *Health Expenditure*, p. 21, table 1.

(10) *Equipment and supplies*: These figures are approximate only. They include the figures given by Deeble for appliances outside hospitals (1974-1975, $71 million; 1975-1976 $81 million in Australian dollars) and an estimate for hospital equipment and supplies at 29 percent of hospital running costs.

(11) *Buildings*: See Deeble, *Health Expenditure*, p. 25, table 4.

Table C-2
Canada
(thousands of Canadian dollars, unless stated otherwise)

	1974	1974 Percentage	1975	1975 Percentage	Notes
Basic data					
1. Population (thousands)	22,395.4		22,726.9		(1)
2. GNP (millions)	147,528		165,428		
3. GNP per capita (dollars)	6,587		7,279		
Health expenditure by source of finance					
4. Public					
(a) General taxation	6,320,829	63.8	7,790,696	66.3	(2)
(b) Public insurance	1,000,086	10.1	1,069,842	9.1	
	7,320,915	73.9	8,860,538	75.4	
4. Public (alternative breakdown)					
(a) Federal	3,137,777	31.7	3,745,523	31.9	
(b) Provincial	4,054,539	40.9	4,975,870	42.3	
(c) Local	128,599	1.3	139,145	1.2	
	7,320,915	73.9	8,860,538	75.4	
5. Consumers					
(a) Private insurance	235,884	2.4	299,147	2.5	(3)
(b) Direct payment	2,043,688	20.6	2,287,725	19.5	
(c) Other	311,801	3.1	301,831	2.6	
	2,591,373	26.1	2,888,703	24.6	
6. Other	—		—		
7. Total expenditures					
(a) Total	9,912,288	100.0	11,749,241	100.0	(4)
(b) Per capita (dollars)	442.60		516.98		
(c) Percentage of GNP	6.7		7.1		
(d) Percentage of GDP	6.6		7.0		
Health expenditure by ownership/administration of channel of provision					
8. Government institutions					
(a) Federal	223,356		246,624		
(b) Provincial	1,025,690		1,236,795		
(c) Local	877,284		950,739		
	2,126,330	21.4	2,434,158	20.7	
9. Nongovernment, not for profit	3,497,302	35.3	4,360,491	37.1	
10. Private, for-profit	4,288,656	43.3	4,954,592	42.2	(5)
11. Other	—		—		
12. Total (8-11)	9,912,288	100.0	11,749,241	100.0	

Table C-2 *(continued)*

	1974	1974 Percentage	1975	1975 Percentage	Notes (1)
Health expenditure by service					
13. Hospitals and homes (current)					
(a) General and allied	3,868,282		4,720,516		
(b) Mental	605,823		704,653		
(c) Tuberculosis	6,412		7,087		
(d) Federal	98,524		101,451		
(e) Homes for special care (nursing homes)	642,760		791,587		
	5,221,801	52.7	6,325,294	53.8	(6)
14. Hospitals (capital)	564,804	5.7	606,102	5.2	(7)
		58.4		59.0	
15. Care by private practitioners					(8)
(a) Primary care	728,973		835,642		
(b) Specialist care	918,052		1,064,841		
(c) Other care	630,635		770,266		
(d) Prescriptions	498,026		573,715		(9)
	2,775,686	28.0	3,244,464	27.6	
(e) Capital	See note 7		See note 7		
16. Self-medication	459,481	4.6	532,356	4.5	(10)
17. Other services					
(a) Public health	317,970	3.2	380,651	3.2	(11)
(b) Research	110,345	1.1	118,827	1.1	(12)
(c) Education	—		—		(13)
18. Administration	172,143	1.7	203,949	1.7	(14)
19. Other	290,058	3.0	337,598	2.9	(15)
20. Total (13-19)	9,912,288	100.0	11,749,241	100.0	

	Cost	Percentage	Number	Cost	Percentage	Number	Notes
Health expenditure by resource							
Manpower							
21. Doctors							
(a) General practice	728,973	7.3	12,426	835,642	7.1	12,911	
(b) All other	1,097,073	11.1	23,110	1,272,830	10.8	24,253	
Dentists							
(a) General practice	431,445	4.4	7,723	531,356	4.5	7,444	
(b) All other	51,198	0.5	596	61,523	0.5	614	
22. Nurses (qualified)			91,737			95,392	(16)
23. Nurses (other)			101,399			101,565	
Total nursing	1,349,915	13.6	193,136	1,677,392	14.3	196,957	
24. Professional and technical	570,530	5.8	57,327	686,895	5.8	59,767	
25. Administrative and clerical and auxiliary	758,459	7.6	113,209	926,899	7.9	106,393	
Mental hospital salaries	436,578	4.4	—	507,335	4.3	—	
26. Total manpower	5,424,171	54.7	407,527	6,499,872	55.3	408,339	(17)

Table C-2 *(continued)*

	1974	1974 Percentage	1975	1975 Percentage	Notes
27. Pharmaceuticals					
(a) Prescribed	597,362	6.0	688,986	5.9	
(b) OTC drugs	459,481	4.7	532,356	4.5	
	1,056,843	10.7	1,221,342	10.4	
28. Equipment and supplies	1,315,451	13.3	1,570,145	13.4	
29. Buildings	564,804	5.7	606,102	5.2	
30. Other	1,551,019	15.6	1,851,780	15.7	(17)
31. Total (21-30)	9,912,288	100.0	11,749,241	100.0	

Source: The Canadian figures were provided by Health and Welfare Canada. I particularly thank W.A. Mennie, director, Health Economics and Data Analysis, for the help given by him and by his staff. The numbered references are to the right-hand column of the Canadian tables.

Reference notes:

(1) *Population*: This figure is derived from a Statistics Canada intercensal estimate, and applies to 1 July of each year.

(2) *Public expenditure*: The great bulk of government expenditure on health services in Canada is financed from general taxation. However, a few provinces collect premiums, and one province has compulsory payroll deduction.

(3) *Payments by consumers*: Direct payment by consumers is arrived at as a residual after deducting other types of finance, including what may be an underestimate of private health insurance. *The latter could in fact be as high as 5 percent of total expenditure, thus reducing direct payment to 17 percent.* "Other" payments by consumers include receipts from charities and voluntary organizations.

(4) *Total health-care expenditure*: As in every other country, the boundary between health-care expenditure and other types of spending (particularly on welfare services and on education) is arbitrary and depends on statistical conventions built up over the years. Nursing homes, homes for the aged, and convalescent homes are financed as health services, as are residential institutions for the mentally ill, the mentally handicapped, alcoholics, and drug addicts. Some community services are excluded where they happen to have been organized by agencies other than hospitals or public-health departments. The cost of health care for the armed forces in hospitals in Canada is included, but not that of any health services overseas or the salaries of medical personnel providing health care outside hospitals. *Almost all education and training for health personnel are excluded from the costs.* Where they are provided within hospitals or as part of in-service government programs, educational expenses are included, but not those for university medical schools or for community colleges (which run most basic nursing courses). *Cash allowances are in all cases excluded from the figures*—a convention I have tried to follow in all the survey countries. In comparison with the other countries, the Canadian figures give, in my opinion, a reasonably comprehensive view of health-care expenditures, with some understatement of spending on educational and community programs. See also table 2-1.

(5) *Private for-profit institutions and contractors*: This includes hospitals and homes for special care (nursing homes) run on a for-profit basis. It also includes the revenue of physicians, dentists, and nurses from private practice; the income of osteopaths and chiropractors; and the revenue of retail pharmacists from the sales of prescribed and nonprescribed drugs.

(6) *Hospital expenditure (current)*: Current operating costs in Canada include amortization, except where the capital cost has been funded directly as capital expenditure. Thus the boundary between capital and current spending is somewhat blurred. Hospital expenditure includes inpatient and outpatient programs, and no breakdown between the two is available nationally. In this analysis, homes for special care (nursing homes) are grouped with hospitals, as shown in the tables.

(7) *Hospital expenditure (capital)*: This includes *all* expenditure on medical facilities construction, including clinics, first-aid stations, sanatoria, and nursing homes.

(8) *Care by private practitioners*: Some hospital expenditure is included here since this covers payments to physicians in private practice, including fees for work done in institutions. All salaried institutional staff are excluded, however.

(9) *Other care*: This represents the aggregate income of dentists, chiropractors, osteopaths, optometrists, podiatrists, private-duty nurses, and the Victorian Order of Nurses from their professional practice.

(10) *Self-medication*: Only the cost of nonprescribed drugs is included here.

(11) *Public health*: Public health covers expenditures by all levels of government for the prevention of disease and protection of health, for the general administration of health departments, and for organizing the delivery of health services. It excludes the administration costs of health-insurance programs.

Table C-2 *(continued)*

(12) *Research*: Health research represents expenditure by government at all levels and by the private sector on investigative activity intended to advance human health, along with related statistical and analytical activity. It excludes research expenditures by pharmaceutical and medical-supply companies, which are charged for in the prices of their products.

(13) *Education*: Education costs are almost all excluded (see note 4). To the extent that they are included (such as those for in-service training programs in hospitals), the costs are included in other items and are not identifiable separately.

(14) *Administration*: The administration costs of health-insurance programs, public and private, are included here, but *not* the costs of administering health programs and institutions. These are, however, included in total expenditure. See also note 11.

(15) *Other*: This category includes occupational-health services, the activities of voluntary health organizations, and a few other miscellaneous items.

(16) *Manpower numbers and costs*: In the case of hospital employees, manpower numbers represent the sum of the number of full-time staff and half the number of part-time staff. *Many health personnel working outside hospitals are excluded because their numbers are not known.* Thus the aggregate numbers shown for Canada represent an underrecording. Manpower costs for mental hospitals are not broken down by manpower category. For doctors and dentists they have been estimated. For other categories of staff (lines 22 to 25) mental-hospital manpower *numbers* are included, with the *costs* shown separately below and added into total manpower costs. To derive costs for table 4-3, I have distributed mental-hospital salaries by calculating an average cost for professional and technical staff from line 24 ($11,500) and for administrative and other staff from line 25 ($8,700) and applying these same rates to the 5,660 professional and technical staff and 11,865 administrative and other staff working in mental hospitals in 1975; I have then assumed that the balance of mental-hospital salaries in 1975 applied to nurses. The resulting percentages of total 1975 costs are 17.1 for nurses, 6.4 for professional and technical, and 8.8 for administrative, clerical, and auxiliary. Different assumptions about the distribution of mental-hospital salaries would result in slightly different figures for these three percentages in table 4-3.

(17) *Other costs and total manpower costs*: The other category (line 30) is a balancing item. Among the components are health research, health administration and prepayment, and the operating cost of homes for special care for which no resource breakdown is available. If, as seems a reasonable assumption, the resource breakdown for these activities is similar to that of other services, then the proportion of total expenditure represented by manpower costs rises to nearly 64 percent.

Table C-3
France
(millions of francs, unless stated otherwise)

	1974	1974 Percentage	1975	1975 Percentage	Notes
Basic data					
1. Population (thousands)	52,491		52,743		(1)
2. GNP (billions of francs)	1,324.8		NA		(2)
GDP (billions of francs)	1,277.6		1,439.0		
3. GNP per capita (francs)	25,239		NA		
GDP per capita (francs)	24,339		27,283		
Health expenditure by source of finance					
4. Public					
(a) General taxation			8,257.8	7.0	
(b) Public insurance-					
social security			80,886.8	69.0	
			89,144.6	76.0	
					(3)
5. Consumers					
(a) Private insurance			3,513.9	3.0	
(b) Direct payment			22,965.4	19.6	
			26,479.3	22.6	
6. Other			1,591.5	1.4	
7. Total expenditure					
(a) Total			117,215.5	100.0	(4)
(b) Per capita (francs)			2,222		
(c) Percentage of GNP			(7.9)		(5)
(d) Percentage of GDP			8.15		
Health expenditure by ownership/administration of channel of provision					
8. Government institutions (state-owned and -run)			43,637	37.2	
9. Nongovernment, not for profit					
10. Private, for-profit institutions and contractors			73,193	62.5	(6)
11. Other (breakdown not available)			385	0.3	
12. Total (8-11)			117,215	100.0	
Health expenditure by service					
13. Hospitals (current)			44,544	38.0	(7)
14. Hospitals (capital)					

Table C-3 *(continued)*

	1974	1974 Percentage	1975	1975 Percentage	Notes
15. Care outside hospitals					
(a) Primary care			52,149	44.5	(8)
(b) Specialist care					
(c) Capital expenditure					
16. Self-Medication			4,507	3.8	
17. Other services					
(a) Public health			1,341	1.1	
(b) Research			1,302	1.1	(9)
(c) Education			1,394	1.2	
(d) Other					
18. Administration			10,875	9.3	(10)
19. Other			1,103	1.0	(11)
20. Total (13-19)			117,215	100.0	

	Cost	Per-centage	Number	Cost	Per-centage	Number
Health expenditure by resource						
Manpower						
21. Doctors						
(a) General practice			46,195	9,162	7.8	48,256
(b) All other			27,357	11,131	9.5	28,887
Total			73,552	20,293	17.3	77,143
Dentists			23,822	8,981	7.7	25,069
22. Nurses (qualified)			182,666			187,531
Midwives			8,374			8,803	(12)
23. Nurses (other)			37,559			40,627
Total nursing			228,599	38,877	33.1	236,961
24. Professional and technical						560,827
25. Administrative and clerical and auxiliary						
26. Total manpower				68,151	58.1	900,000

	1974	1974 Percentage	1975	1975 Percentage	
27. Pharmaceuticals					
(a) Prescribed	17,214		20,263	17.3	
(b) OTC drugs	3,779		4,353	3.7	(13)
	20,993		24,616	21.0	
28. Equipment and supplies					
			22,769	19.5	(14)
29. Buildings					
30. Other			1,679	1.4	(15)
31. Total (21-30)			117,215	100.0	

Table C-3 *(continued)*

Source: The acknowledged center for information on health expenditures in France is CREDOC (Centre de recherche pour l'étude et l'observation des conditions de vie), an independent, publicly funded research center in Paris. The main source for the figures that follow is CREDOC's *La Dépense Nationale de Santé en 1975* in its series on national accounts. Madame Sandier and her colleagues at CREDOC helped me to understand the data, and I gladly acknowledge my debt to them. Care must be taken in comparing these figures with others attributed to CREDOC in various international publications. The CREDOC figures usually quoted are for *consommation médicale finale*, which is a relatively narrow definition, excluding teaching, research, preventive-health activities, and administration. In 1975, for example, *consommation médicale finale* represented 85.5 percent of *dépense nationale de santé*, the definition that I have used. 1974 figures have not been published in comparable form. The references are to the right-hand column of the French tables.

NA = not available.

Reference notes:

(1) *Population*: The population figures are mid-year estimates.

(2) *GNP/GDP*: France may have ceased calculating GNP figures, as opposed to GDP. In 1974, the latest year for which GNP figures were available, GDP represented 96.4 percent of GNP.

(3) *Expenditure by source of finance*: These figures can be found in table 2 on page 12 of *La Dépense Nationale de Santé en 1975*, which also gives a breakdown by service. The heading "other" (line 6) covers employers (1.2 percent of total expenditure) and voluntary and professional organizations like the Red Cross (0.2 percent of total expenditure).

(4) *Total expenditure*: The total appears comprehensive in comparison with those for other countries. For example, education costs *include university preclinical education* for doctors and other members of the health professions. An attempt has also been made to include all research costs. The latter are shown as gross figures, and also net of double counting, eliminating expenditures financed by charges elsewhere in the system, such as research financed by the drug companies and recovered by them from drug sales. The net figures for research expenditure are used in this analysis. Administration costs are included for government and for the health-insurance agencies, as well as for hospitals. Travel costs are included to the extent that they are reimbursed by health insurance or borne directly by public agencies. (However, total transport costs represent only 0.6 percent of total health-care expenditures for France.) As in other countries, the main area of uncertainty concerns the boundary between health and welfare expenditures for services for the elderly, the handicapped, the mentally ill, and similar groups. Broadly speaking, medical-type institutions are included and all others excluded, so that the boundary depends on the classification of the agency concerned. The French have institutions for physically and mentally handicapped children that are considered part of the health system but would not be so considered in some other countries, such as Australia. See also table 2-1.

(5) *Percentage of GNP*: This is estimated from GDP, using the 1974 relationship between the two (see note 2).

(6) *Expenditure by ownership/administration*: This breakdown is not wholly available from the CREDOC publication. I have estimated it from that source (particularly tables 10, 14, and 19) with help from CREDOC staff:

	Public (Millions of francs)	Private (Including Nonprofit) (Millions of francs)
Hospital services	28,374	15,952
Education	1,314	80
Research	1,194	108
Prevention	1,341	—
Administration	10,005	870
Health services outside hospitals	766	29,875
Medical supplies	—	24,312
Transport	—	717
Transfers	643	1
Services provided by companies	—	1,278
	43,637	73,193

Within the private sector, the split between nonprofit and profit is never an easy one to make. By analogy from other countries, the following can be allocated to one or the other:

Table C-3 *(continued)*

	Private Nonprofit (Millions of francs)	Private for Profit (Millions of francs)
Private practice of doctors, dentists and others		28,105
Medical supplies		24,312
Education	80	—
Research	108	—
	188	52,417
Percentage of total health-care expenditure	1.6	44.7

A minimum of 44.7 percent of total expenditure can, on this basis, be classified as being run for profit, and 1.6 percent as nonprofit, with the balance of 16.2 percent being doubtful. The main uncertainty concerns the classification of nongovernment hospital services (13.6 percent of total expenditures).

(7) *Hospital expenditure*: Line 13 includes *inpatient care only*. Ambulatory care, even when linked to hospitals, is included in line 15. For hospital costs no breakdown is available between running expenses and capital expenditure. The latter is included in private hospital costs by means of a 5.5 percent amortization charge.

(8) *Care outside hospitals*: This line includes the costs of hospital outpatient services, as well as of home care. Unfortunately, no breakdown is available between the two. The total comprises (from the CREDOC publication, table 10):

	Millions of Francs	
Physicians' fees	16,188	
Laboratory analyses	2,480	
Auxiliaries' fees (nurses, midwives and so on)	3,761	
Dentists' fees	8,981	
Spas	577	
Rehabilitation	322	
Ambulatory care (excluding medical supplies)		32,309
Drugs (less self-medication, line 16)	18,029	
Eyeglasses, hearing aids, and so on	1,811	
Medical supplies		19,840
		52,149

(9) *Other services*: For details see the CREDOC publication, tables 14 to 18.

(10) *Administration*: The makeup of this figure (from table 19 of the CREDOC publication) is:

	Millions of Francs
Government	448
Social security (proportional to health's share of total premium income)	9,556
Insurance companies	665
Other (including voluntary and professional organizations)	206
	10,875

(11) *Other*: This line includes transport (717 million francs) and line 11 (385 million francs).

(12) *Manpower numbers and costs*: These figures are estimated with the help of CREDOC but do not appear in *La Dépense Nationale de Santé en 1975*. Manpower numbers are from national statistics; the total of 900,000 is not an exact figure. Manpower costs were obtained by combining known figures with estimates based on percentages from social-security records. For example, in the case of physicians:

Table C-3 *(continued)*

	Millions of Francs
Physicians' fees for ambulatory and home care (see note 8)	16,188
Physicians' fees for hospital care	
70 percent of fees from public hospitals = 70/100 × 1,870 =	1,309
91 percent of fees from private hospitals = 91/100 × 3,072 =	2,796
	20,293

The breakdown of this total between generalists and specialists was estimated as:

Generalists: 56.6 percent x fees for ambulatory and home care = 56.6/100 × 16,188 =	9,162
Specialists: 43.4 percent × these fees = 43.4/100 × 16,188 =	7,026
Hospital fees as previously shown	{ 1,309
	{ 2,796
	11,131

The calculation for total personnel costs was:

		Millions of Francs
60 percent of hospital costs after deducting physicians' fees = 60/100 × [44,544 − (1,870 + 3,072)] =		23,761
Auxiliaries' fees (as in note 8)	3,761	
1 percent of physicians' fees in public hospitals	19	
3 percent of physicians' fees in private hospitals	92	3,872
Administration salaries (CREDOC, table 12)		6,155
74 percent of education costs = 74/100 × 1,394 =		1,031
74 percent of research costs = 74/100 × 1,302 =		963
100 percent of rehabilitation costs		322
70 percent of public-health costs = 70/100 × 1,341 =		939
60 percent of laboratory analysis costs = 60/100 × 2,480 =		1,488
60 percent of costs of spas = 60/100 × 577 =		346
		38,877
Dentists (CREDOC, table 10)		8,981
Physicians (as previously shown)		20,293
		68,151

(13) *Pharmaceutical costs*: The source of these figures is another CREDOC study *La Pharmacie dans le Système de Santé Suède/France*, 1977. See pp. 146-149, tables C.5-C.9.

(14) *Equipment, supplies, and buildings*: These costs are derived as a residual.

(15) *Other*: These costs comprise:

	Millions of Francs
Transport	717
Spas	577
No breakdown available (line 11)	385
	1,679

Table C-4
West Germany
(millions of Deutschmarks, unless stated otherwise)

	1974	1974 Percentage	1975	1975 Percentage	Notes
Basic data					
1. Population (thousands)	62,054		61,829		
2. GNP	986,900		1,030,300		
GDP	987,100		1,029,400		
3. GNP per capita					
(Deutschmarks)	15,904		16,663		
GDP per capita					
(Deutschmarks)	15,907		16,649		
Health expenditure by source of finance					
4. Public					
(a) General taxation	13,260	15.6	14,199	14.6	
(b) Public insurance-					
social security	51,824	61.0	60,751	62.5	(1)
	65,084	76.6	74,950	77.1	
5. Consumers					
(a) Private insurance	4,799	5.6	5,133	5.3	(1)
(b) Direct payment	10,769	12.7	12,108	12.5	
	15,568	18.3	17,241	17.8	
6. Other—Employers					
(direct)	4,314	5.1	4,935	5.1	
7. Total expenditure					
(a) Total	84,966	100.0	97,126	100.0	(2)
(b) Per capita					
(Deutschmarks)	1,369		1,571		
(c) Percentage of GNP	8.6		9.4		
(d) Percentage of GDP	8.6		9.4		
Health expenditure by ownership/administration of channel of provision					
8. Government institutions					
(state-owned and -run)			19,363	19.9	
9. Nongovernment, not for					
profit					
			77,763	80.1	(3)
10. Private, for-profit					
institutions and					
contractors					
11. Other			—	—	
12. Total (8-11)	84,966	100.0	97,126	100.0	
Health expenditure by service					
13. Hospitals (current)	26,992	31.8	30,586	31.5	(4)
14. Hospitals (capital)	3,344	3.9	3,365	3.5	(5)
	30,336	35.7	33,951	35.0	

Table C-4 *(continued)*

	1974	1974 Percentage	1975	1975 Percentage	Notes
15. Care outside hospitals, including private physicians' fees for hospital care	25,691	30.2	29,345	30.2	(4)
16. Self-medication	3,892	4.6	4,379	4.5	
17. Other services					
(a) Public health	2,964	3.5	3,150	3.2	
(b) Research	227	0.3	288	0.3	(6)
(c) Education	1,597	1.9	1,699	1.7	(6)
(d) Diagnosis and surveillance	4,491	5.3	5,331	5.5	(7)
(e) Rehabilitation services	1,619	1.9	1,909	2.0	
(f) False teeth	4,329	5.1	6,454	6.6	
(g) Spa treatment	4,494	5.3	4,832	5.0	
18. Administration	5,326	6.2	5,788	6.0	(8)
19. Other	—		—		
20. Total (13-19)	84,966	100.0	97,126	100.0	

	Cost	Per- centage	Number	Cost	Per- centage	Number	
Health expenditure by resource							
21. Doctors							
(a) General practice			64,137			64,627	
(b) All other			50,524			54,099	
			114,661			118,726	
Dentists			31,538			31,774	
22. Nurses (qualified)			216,457			229,590	
23. Nurses (other)			40,130			37,991	(9)
Total nursing			256,587			267,581	(10)
24. Profession and technical							
(a) Pharmacists			24,787			25,597	
(b) Other medical and technical			75,396			78,733	
(c) Educational			5,173			5,393	(9)
			105,356			109,723	(10)
25. Administrative and clerical			48,326			49,536	(9)
and auxiliary			194,668			194,535	(9)
			242,994			244,071	(9)
26. Total manpower	?	?	751,136	?	?	771,875	(10)
27. Pharmaceuticals							
(a) Prescribed	11,327	13.3		12,967	13.4		
(b) OTC drugs	3,892	4.6		4,379	4.5		
	15,219	17.9		17,346	17.9		
28. Equipment and supplies							
(a) False teeth	4,329	5.1		6,454	6.6		
(b) Other	?	?		?	?		
29. Buildings and other capital	4,481	5.2		4,463	4.6		
30. Other—subsidiaries	1,022	1.2		1,052	1.1		(11)
31. Total (21-30)	84,966	100.0		97,126	100.0		

Table C-4 *(continued)*

Source: The German figures are principally based on *Die Struktur der Ausgaben im Gesundheitsbereich und ihre Entwicklung seit 1970*, prepared by the Federal Government Statistics Office, Statistisches Bundesamt. I am grateful to Dr. H. Essig and Herr Müller for their help in extracting and interpreting the figures which I needed. The numbered references are to the right-hand column of the German tables.

Reference notes:

(1) *The role of employers*: Public and private employers play a major role in financing health care in Germany, through the compulsory and voluntary insurance schemes. Almost 50 percent of the total bill for health services is met by employers' contributions.

(2) *Total health-care expenditure*: The total is as given in the Statistisches Bundesamt report, less all cash benefits. (I have not, however, made any reduction in the administration costs recorded for Germany. A pro-rata reduction in administration costs attributable to health-insurance organizations might lower total health-care spending by 1 percent.) This total parallels my interpretation of the figures for other countries, where I have similarly excluded cash benefits. Total health-care expenditures for Germany are among the highest in the world in terms of GNP—a finding also arrived at by U.E. Reinhardt in *National Health Insurance: A Synopsis* (prepared for National Center for Health Services Research, Washington, 1977). This high spending does not seem to be accounted for by differences in definition, once cash benefits are excluded. For example, the Federal Republic, like other countries, generally includes in health expenditures only those activities that are managed by a health agency or reimbursed under health legislation or health insurance. This leaves out community programs conventionally viewed as the concern of other, nonhealth agencies. Similarly, some health services for the armed forces and for prisoners are excluded, as are transport costs when not met by government or by insurance companies. Administration costs are included only in relation to health insurance (public and private) and health agencies, not in relation to government or employers. Some costs are undoubtedly higher in Germany than elsewhere, such as treatment at health spas (5 percent of total expenditure in 1975) and, apparently, the cost of false teeth (6.5 percent of total expenditure in that year). For overall comparability see also table 2-1.

(3) *Ownership and administration*: Expenditure in government institutions is estimated as follows for 1975:

	Millions of Deutschmarks
Public hospitals (representing 54 percent of total beds)	14,832
Rehabilitation services in public institutions	694
Education and research	1,987
Preventive and other public programs (public health, social medicine, and so on)	1,850
	19,363

19,363 Deutschmarks represents 19.9 percent of total health-care expenditure. For the balance, no breakdown is available between for-profit and nonprofit.

(4) *Hospital current expenditure*: My estimate includes all costs of *stationäre behandlung* (inpatient treatment) plus half the total cost of prescribed drugs. Unfortunately, as in the United States and some other countries, this excludes from hospital expenditures substantial fees paid to private physicians for attendance on hospital patients. These, however, are included in line 15 and hence in total expenditure.

(5) *Hospital capital expenditure*: In addition to *hospital* capital expenditures, roughly another 1,000 million Deutschmarks was spent in both 1974 and 1975 on capital projects for other health purposes, such as health spas, education, research, public health, and health administration. These nonhospital capital expenditures are included in the cost of the service concerned in lines 17 to 18, but can be separately identified in the original German publication, and are grouped with hospital capital expenditure in line 29.

(6) *Research and education*: As is so often the case with national accounts, the demarcation reflects organizational boundaries rather than activities. In the German definition, education expenditures include medical research in universities, and the research item (line 17b) is for research in places outside university medical centers. On the other hand, a substantial amount of educational expenditure, such as that for nurses, is included elsewhere in this table, rather than in line 17c.

(7) *Diagnosis and surveillance*: Line 17d has no exact parallel in the accounts for any other country. It comprises preventive activities outside the traditional definition of public health, particularly where these activities are paid for by the insurance companies.

(8) *Administration*: This item excludes the costs of government administration (such as the ministry of health) and of hospitals and other health agencies. It reflects the cost of running the health-insurance system.

(9) and (10) *Manpower numbers*: The principal source for these figures is the *Statistisches Jahrbuch 1977 für die Bundesrepublik Deutschland*. Items marked (9) are for *hospital* personnel only, and hence items marked (10) are in-

Table C-4 *(continued)*

complete since they exclude some people working in community-based health programs. Unfortunately, I have been unable to obtain any authoritative estimate of health-manpower costs for Germany. By deduction, and estimating line 28b at 10-12 percent of total expenditure, one reaches a "guesstimate" for health-manpower costs of 58-60 percent of total health-care expenditures. This is similar to that for other countries.

(11) *Subsidies*: This line represents subsidies paid by government and insurers to private institutions, presumably to help meet deficits.

Table C-5
Italy
(thousand million Italian lire, unless stated otherwise)

	1974	1974 Percentage	1975	1975 Percentage	Notes
Basic data					
1. Population (thousands)	55,412		55,830		(1)
2. GNP per capita	101,541		114,530		
GDP per capita	101,723		115,072		
3. GNP per capita					
(million lire)	1.832		2.051		
GDP per capita					
(million lire)	1.836		2.061		
Health expenditure by source of finance					
4. Public					
(a) General taxation	844	12.4	1,947	23.8	(2)
(b) Compulsory insur-					
ance-social security	5,209	76.2	5,509	67.5	(2) and (3)
	6,053	88.6	7,456	91.3	
5. Consumers					
(a) Private insurance	780	11.4	710	8.7	
(b) Direct payment					
6. Other (specify)	—		—		
7. Total expenditure					
(a) Total	6,833	100.0	8,166	100.0	(4)
(b) Per capita (thousand					
lire)	123.313		146.265		
(c) Percentage of GNP	6.73		7.13		
(d) Percentage of GDP	6.72		7.10		
Health expenditure by ownership/administration of channel of provision					
8. Government institutions					
(state-owned and -run)			4,945	60.6	
9. Nongovernment, not for					(5)
profit			3,221	39.4	
10. Private, for-profit					
institutions and					
contractors					
11. Other					
12. Total (8-11)	6,833	100.0	8,166	100.0	
Health expenditure by service					
13. Hospitals (current)					
	3,380	49.5	3,918	48.0	(6)
14. Hospitals (capital)					
15. Care outside hospitals					
(a) Primary care					
(b) Specialist care	2,247	32.9	2,846	34.9	(7)
(c) Capital expenditure	—	—	—	—	

Table C-5 *(continued)*

	1974	1974 Percentage	1975	1975 Percentage	Notes
16. Self-Medication	430	6.3	460	5.6	(8)
17. Other services					
(a) Public health	162	2.4	184	2.2	
(b) Research					
(c) Education	—		—		
(d) Other	179	2.6	239	2.9	
18. Administration	435	6.3	519	6.4	(9)
19. Other	—		—		
20. Total (13-19)	6,833	100.0	8,166	100.0	

		1975		
	Cost	Percentage of Total Cost	Number	Notes
Health expenditure by resource				
Manpower				
21. Doctors	1,900	23.3	111,110	
(a) General practitioners			43,200	
(b) Dentists			7,600	(+3,000 general practitioners
(c) All other			60,310	practicing dentistry)
22. Nurses (qualified)			85,487	
(a) In hospitals			67,327	
(b) Community			11,160	(midwives)
(c) Social security institutions			7,000	
23. Nurses (other)			124,579	
(a) In hospitals			118,079	
(b) Community			4,500	
(c) Social security institutions			2,000	
Total nursing	1,301	15.9	210,066	
24. Professional and technical	201	2.5	59,028	
(a) In hospitals			17,728	
(b) Social security institutions			4,300	
(c) Pharmacists			37,000	
25. Administrative and clerical and auxiliary	1,241	15.2	247,970	
(a) Administrative and clerical in hospitals			35,275	
(b) Administrative and clerical in social security institutions			31,117	
(c) Works and maintenance staff in hospital			62,602	
(d) Auxiliaries in hospitals			118,976	
26. Total manpower	4,643	56.9	628,174	
(a) Working in public institutions			495,883	
(b) Working in private institutions or as professionals			132,291	

(10)

Table C-5 *(continued)*

	1974	1974 Percentage	1975	1975 Percentage	Notes
27. Pharmaceuticals					
(a) Prescribed	930	13.6	1,179	14.4	(11)
(b) OTC drugs	430	6.3	460	5.6	
	1,360	19.9	1,639	20.0	
28. Equipment and supplies			1,884	23.1	(12)
29. Buildings					
30. Other					
31. Total (21-30)	6,833	100.0	8,166	100.0	

Source: Obtaining reliable, reasonably complete health expenditure data for Italy poses even more formidable difficulties than for other countries. Until very recently the accounts of the social-insurance funds (particularly INAM) have been virtually the only information source, and these accounts have to be studied against the background of Italian events and laws, with their rather special flavor. For example, after the Hospital Reform of 1968, hospitals were entitled by law to charge the insurance companies a price per day calculated from their total costs divided by their bed days. The companies could not contest this price, but on the other hand their income (also set by law) did not keep pace with it. The insurance companies therefore could not pay the hospitals. Notwithstanding that their income and expenditure balanced on paper, the hospitals could not pay their suppliers and were forced to borrow from the banks to pay their staff. Before the new reform went into effect in 1975, the hospitals had not paid some suppliers for more than a year. And in 1974 the health sector incurred interest charges of an estimated 535 thousand million lire, equivalent to roughly 7 percent of total expenditure. For both 1974 and 1975 interest charges have been excluded from the figures given on the grounds that they represent a cost of government borrowing rather than an internationally comparable cost of supplying health services.

I am deeply indebted for the Italian part of my analysis to Professor Antonio Brenna and Dr. Vittorio Mapelli, at the Instituto per la ricerca di Economia Sanitaria in Milan. The data are based on their research.

References are to the numbers in the right hand column of the Italian tables.

Reference notes:

(1) *Population*: The population figures for each year are derived from the average of the figures for 1 January of that year and 1 January of the following year, as given in the national statistics.

(2) *General taxation and public insurance*: The change, from 1974 to 1975, in the balance between public-insurance and general-tax funding is accounted for by the reform, which went into effect on 1 January 1975. From that date, central government became responsible for financing the general hospitals by means of a new public fund. This fund drew just under two-thirds of its income from social insurance and the remainder direct from the Treasury.

(3) *Public insurance*: This figure (in line with those for the other nine countries) excludes cash allowances paid as sickness benefits. It also excludes interest.

(4) *Total expenditure*: The overall estimate for Italian health-care expenditure is likely to be too low rather than too high, given the fragmentary nature of the data sources and the confusion of the system. In addition some spending classed as health-care expenditure in at least some of the other countries is viewed as social expenditure in Italy (for example, services for the mentally and physically handicapped and for alcoholics and drug addicts). Among education costs, university costs for the preclinical training of doctors, dentists, and pharmacists are excluded from health-care expenditure. Travel costs include ambulance costs only. Administration costs include figures for the central ministry of health and for the regions but not for local government. For the social-insurance funds, administrative costs are included in part, after an estimate of the costs relating to sickness benefits is deducted. Research costs are chiefly those related to research in hospitals, and even then exclude funding from nonpublic sources. See also table 2-1 for Italy's comparability to other countries.

(5) *Ownership and administration*: Line 8 includes public hospitals and all activities run directly by government at any level or by the social-security system.

(6) *Hospital expenditure*: Capital costs are mainly included by means of an amortization charge, rather than at the time of construction. The amortization period is up to twenty-five years, plus interest at the actual rate incurred.

(7) *Care outside hospitals*: These figures include:

Table C-5 *(continued)*

	1974	1975
	(thousand million lire)	
General-practitioner services	759	948
Specialist services	558	719
Pharmaceuticals prescribed	930	1,179
	2,247	2,846

(8) *Self-medication*: This is the estimated cost of pharmaceuticals not reimbursed from public funds. It is thus an overestimate for self-medication, since it includes nonreimbursed costs of prescribed drugs.

(9) *Administrative costs*: For the definition of administrative costs (which is a comprehensive one, above the local level) see note 4.

(10) *Manpower numbers and costs*: Manpower figures are fragmentary, and manpower costs are estimated from incomplete information.

(11) *Pharmaceuticals*: The costs given do not include drugs prescribed in hospitals and are therefore an underestimate. Hospital drug costs are, however, included in total expenditure.

(12) *Equipment, supplies, and buildings*: This line is estimated as a residual. It includes hospital drugs and medical supplies (see note 11) costing 422 thousand million lire. Unfortunately, the drugs element cannot be separated from medical supplies.

Table C-6
The Netherlands
(millions of guilders, unless stated otherwise)

	1974	1974 Percentage	1975	1975 Percentage	Notes
Basic data					
1. Population (thousands)	13,545		13,667		(1)
2. GNP	191,340		207,780		
GDP	190,290		208,930		
3. GNP per capita (guilders)	14,126		15,203		
GDP per capita (guilders)	14,049		15,287		
Health expenditure by source of finance					
4. Public					
(a) General taxation	2,229.3	15.1			(2)
(b) Public insurance-					
social security	8,270.1	56.0			(3)
		71.1			
5. Consumers					
(a) Private insurance	} 4,038.5	27.3			(4)
(b) Direct payment					
6. Other	233.4	1.6			(4)
7. Total expenditure					
(a) Total	14,771.3				(5)
(b) Per capita	1,091				
(c) Percentage of GNP	7.72				
(d) Percentage of GDP	7.76				
Health expenditure by ownership/administration of channel of provision					
8. Government institutions (state-owned and -run)	1,550.0	10.5			
9. Nongovernment, not for profit	8,231.4	55.7			(6)
10. Private, for-profit institutions and contractors	4,989.9	33.8			(7)
11. Other	—	—			
12. Total (8-11)	14,771.3	100.0			
Health expenditure by service					
13. Hospitals (current)	6,669.2	45.2			(8)
14. Hospitals (capital)	1,100.0	7.4			(9)
	7,769.2	52.6			

Table C-6 *(continued)*

	1974	1974 Percentage	1975	1975 Percentage	Notes
15. Care outside hospitals (a) Primary care (b) Specialist care (c) Capital expenditure	6,192.4	41.9			(10)
16. Self-medication	NA				
17. Other services (a) Public health (b) Research (c) Education (d) Other	159.1	1.1			
18. Administration	650.6	4.4			(11)
19. Other					
20. Total (13-19)	14,771.3	100.0			

	Cost	Per-centage	Number	Cost	Per-centage	Number

Health Expenditure by resource

Manpower

	Cost	Per-centage	Number	Cost	Per-centage	Number	
21. Doctors (a) General practice (b) All other	2,511.0	17.0	(4,800) (15,500) (20,300)			(4,900) (16,000) (20,900)	(12)
Dentists (a) General practice (b) All other	733.0	5.0	(4,100)			(4,200)	
22. Nurses (qualified)			43,690			47,140	
23. Nurses (other) Total nursing			54,100 97,790			54,700 101,840	(13)
24. Profession and technical			26,190			28,670	
25. Administrative and clerical and auxiliary			67,130			69,610	
26. Total manpower			(215,510)			(225,220)	(13)

	1974	1974 Percentage	1975	1975 Percentage	
27. Pharmaceuticals (a) Prescribed (b) OTC drugs	2,107	14.3 not available & not included			(14)
28. Equipment and supplies					(15)
29. Buildings	1,100.0	7.4	1,285		(16)
30. Other					
31. Total (21-30)	14,771.3	100.0			

Table C-6 *(continued)*

Source: The figures for the Netherlands are based on statistics from the Ministry of Health and Environmental Protection, obtained with the help of Dr. F.F.H. Rutten. I am most grateful to him and to Dr. P. Siderius, the secretary general at the ministry, for their interest in the project. Numbered references correspond to the numbers in the right-hand column of the tables for the Netherlands.

NA = not available.

Reference notes:

(1) *Population*: Mid-year estimates based on end-year population figures from national statistics.

(2) *General taxation*: Of the expenditure from general tax revenue in 1974, 1,208.8 million guilders was contributed to the following social-security funds:

	Millions of Guilders
Health insurance for the elderly	378.6
Voluntary public insurance	41.8
Exceptional Medical Expense Act fund (which covers long-term care)	788.4
	1,208.8

The general tax revenue (2,229.3 million guilders) is all raised by the central government.

(3) *Public insurance*: The makeup of this figure is:

	Millions of Guilders
Compulsory insurance premiums	4,664.1
Insurance for the elderly premiums	442.2
Voluntary public-insurance premiums	849.8
Premiums to the Exceptional Medical Expense Act fund	2,490.8
	8,446.9
Less credits	176.8
	8,270.1

(4) *Payments by consumers and others*: Line 5, which includes private insurance, is based on information from the private insurance companies and should be considered very rough. Other payments, in line 6, represent financing by companies.

(5) *Total expenditure*: Dutch definitions of health-care expenditure seem less bounded by institutional definitions than those of most other countries. Presumably the unparalleled range of institutional forms, and the low share of services actually administered by government (see line 8 in the table), soften the importance of institutional boundaries and turn attention more towards programs. It is therefore not surprising that the Dutch attempt to analyze expenditure by population and disease group, as well as by service—an attempt that is likely to be repeated elsewhere.

There are nevertheless some major omissions from the Dutch figures, which suggest that total expenditure is understated. The principal omissions are: (1) self-medication, which accounts for 4 to 5 percent of total health-care expenditure in most of the other countries surveyed; (2) education at schools and colleges, including nursing education when conducted away from hospitals (clinical and other on-the-job training is included in costs); and (3) medical research, except when paid for by government in financing hospitals. The understatement relative to other countries in this survey might be of the order of 0.4 percent of GNP (5 percent of health-care expenditures).

(6) *Government and nonprofit institutions*: The division between lines 8 and 9 is approximate. The government owns few ambulatory care institutions. It owns about 16 percent of hospitals, including the large, costly university hospitals. These hospitals account for about 20 percent of hospital expenditure, which in turn represents 52.6 percent of total expenditure (see lines 13 and 14).

$$20/100 \times 52.6/100 = 10.5 \text{ percent approximately}$$

Nongovernment public institutions are a special feature of life in the Netherlands, giving to the educational, health, and social services a distinctively decentralized, and at times eccentric, flavor.

Table C-6 *(continued)*

(7) *Private, for-profit*: This sector includes the private practices of physicians, dentists, nurses, and pharmacists.

(8) *Hospital expenditure (current)*: Hospital expenditure covers primarily *inpatient* care, with some polyclinic care when this is linked to hospitals. Hospital expenditure excludes physicians' fees, except when (as in the university hospitals) hospital prices include these fees. About 24 percent of all specialist physicians are salaried, and their costs would be included. For other specialists it is impossible to make any accurate distinction between payments for ambulatory care and those for inpatient care. Thus their fees would all be included in line 15. The breakdown of the hospital expenditure figure is:

	Millions of Guilders
General hospitals	3,434.2
University hospitals	832.4
Specialized hospitals	325.3
Mental hospitals	893.4
Institutions for the mentally handicapped	766.9
Nursing homes	1,334.8
Homes	136.6
Other institutions	45.6
Total	7,769.2
Less amortization (approximate)	1,100.0
Running costs less amortization	6,669.2

(9) *Hospital expenditure (capital)*: Derived from the annual amortization provision (see note 8). In the Netherlands capital construction is generally reimbursed by amortization (over a thirty-year period for buildings) or by inclusion in tariffs and fees. Amortization is based on historic cost.

(10) *Care outside hospitals*: As noted above (note 8) this item includes physicians' fees for inpatient care, except where these fees are included in hospital prices. Included here are the following:

	Millions of Guilders
Physicians' fees	2,311.0
Dentists' fees	733.0
Fees to midwives and paramedical workers	259.0
Pharmacies	1,686.9
The Cross associations	248.9
Maternity-care centers	104.8
School health services	94.3
Other institutions for general social health care	328.0
Child-guidance clinics	29.2
Social-psychiatric services	63.4
Centers for alcoholics and drug addicts	12.3
Other institutions for mental social health care	29.5
Other ambulatory-care institutions	292.1
	6,192.4

(11) *Administration*: The definition of administrative costs is a broad one, including, for example, ministry of health costs and the administrative costs of health insurance. Hospital-administration costs are included in line 13.

(12) *Doctors' costs and numbers*: Physicians' fees are known to be 2,311 million guilders for ambulatory and inpatient care, except where included in hospital prices. Medical salaries included in hospital costs are estimated by me as approximately 200 million guilders, based on partial figures for 1974 and a 1975 figure of 241 million guilders. 2,311 + 200 = 2,511 million guilders. Physician and dentist numbers are estimated from the *Netherlands Compendium of Health Statistics, 1974* (which has 1972 figures in detail) and WHO statistics for 1974.

Table C-6 *(continued)*

(13) *Manpower numbers*: Except for physicians and dentists, numbers are for hospital personnel only and *totals are therefore incomplete*. No reliable estimates are available for manpower (other than physicians and dentists) in community health services.

(14) *Pharmaceutical costs*: For ambulatory care, pharmaceutical costs were 1,687 million guilders in 1974. To this I have added 420 million guilders for drugs and dressings (medical supplies) in hospitals. This is derived from incomplete figures for 1974 and complete figures for 1975 (497 million guilders).

(15) *Equipment and supplies*: Only hospital figures are available, and these are incomplete for 1974. For 1975, equipment and supply costs (including food, energy, equipment and maintenance, and other outside services) accounted for 13.2 percent of hospital costs.

(16) *Buildings*: This figure includes hospital amortization only (see line 14 and note 9).

Table C-7
Sweden
(millions of kronor, unless stated otherwise)

	1974	1974 Percentage	1975	1975 Percentage	Notes
Basic data					
1. Population (thousands)	8,161		8,193		(1)
2. GNP	248,637		286,899		
GDP	248,593		287,078		
3. GNP per capita (kronor)	30,470		35,020		
GDP per capita (kronor)	30,461		35,039		
Health expenditure by source of finance					
4. Public					
(a) General taxation	15,559	77.5	19,145	78.5	(2)
(b) Public insurance—					
social security	2,562	12.8	3,192	13.1	(3)
	18,121	90.3	22,337	91.6	
5. Consumers					
(a) Private insurance	—		—		
(b) Direct payment	1,949	9.7	2,059	8.4	(4)
6. Other	—		—		
7. Total expenditure					
(a) Total	20,070	100.0	24,396	100.0	(5)
(b) Per capita (kronor)	2,459		2,978		
(c) Percentage of GNP	8.1		8.5		
(d) Percentage of GDP	8.1		8.5		
Health expenditure by ownership/administration of channel of provision					
8. Government institutions (state-owned and -run)	16,458	82.0	20,122	82.5	(6)
9. Nongovernment, not for profit	Negligible	—	Negligible	—	
10. Private, for-profit institutions and contractors	3,612	18.0	4,274	17.5	(6)
11. Other	—	—	—	—	
12. Total (8-11)	20,070	100.0	24,396	100.0	
Health expenditure by service					
13. Hospitals (current)	12,726	63.4	15,657	64.1	
14. Hospitals (capital)	1,397	7.0	1,707	7.0	
	14,129	70.4	17,364	71.1	
15. Care outside hospitals	5,083	25.3	5,996	24.6	(7)
16. Self-medication	693	3.5	848	3.5	

Table C-7 *(continued)*

	1974	1974 Percentage	1975	1975 Percentage	Notes
17. Other services					
(a) Public health					
(b) Research	87	0.4	94	0.4	(8)
(c) Education					
(d) Other					
18. Administration	84	0.4	94	0.4	(9)
19. Other	—		—		
20. Total (13-19)	20,070	100.0	24,396	100.0	

	Cost	Per-centage	Number	Cost	Per-centage	Number
Health expenditure by resource						
Manpower						
21. Doctors						
(a) General practice			13,260			14,050
(b) All other						
Dentists						
(a) General practice			7,180			7,060
(b) All other						
22. Nurses (qualified)			47,800			48,380
23. Nurses (other)			(95,000)			(95,000)
Total nursing			(142,800)			(143,380)
24. Professional and technical			(31,000)			(32,000)
25. Administrative and clerical and auxiliary			(110,060)			(124,110)
26. Total manpower	11,567	57.6	304,300	14,273	58.5	320,600

(10)

	1974	1974 Percentage	1975	1975 Percentage	Notes
27. Pharmaceuticals					
(a) Prescribed	1,199	5.9	1,355	5.5	
(b) OTC drugs	693	3.5	848	3.5	
	1,892	9.4	2,203	9.0	
28. Equipment and supplies and other	5,214	26.0	6,213	25.5	(11)
29. Buildings	1,397	7.0	1,707	7.0	(12)
30. Other	—		—		
31. Total (21-30)	20,070	100.0	24,396	100.0	

Source: The figures for Sweden were prepared with the help of the Central Bureau of Statistics and the National Board of Health and Welfare. They are based on the National Accounts, as published in *Statistical Reports* N1978:8.4. I am particularly grateful to Mr. Jan Redeby of the Central Bureau for his assistance. The numbered references are to the right-hand column of the Swedish tables.

Reference notes:

(1) *Population*: Population is the average for the year in question.

(2) *General taxation*: This money is raised very largely by the twenty-five county councils which, along with the city councils of Gothenberg and Malmo, are principally responsible for hospital services in Sweden. Tax levied by the county councils is proportional to income rather than progressive. Spending on health care represents nearly 90 percent of

Table C-7 *(continued)*

county-council expenditure, and is thus the dominant item in county-council budgets. The central government itself contributes a small part of the total from general tax revenues, partly to finance certain national hospitals and partly by way of grants to the county councils.

(3) *Compulsory insurance*: Under the Swedish national health-insurance plan certain medical costs are reimbursed, and cash allowances have been excluded from this tabulation. The fees reimbursed under the insurance plan are primarily for ambulatory cases, including contributions towards the fees of private physicians. A daily fee is also paid to the hospital concerned for inpatient care, but this represents only a fraction of the cost.

(4) *Direct payment by consumers*: These represent payments by households for physicians' fees, dental care, medicines, and so on, after deducting costs reimbursed through the national health-insurance plan (line 4b in the tabulation and note 3).

(5) *Total expenditure*: The definition of health-care expenditures is a reasonably comprehensive one in Sweden, but nevertheless (as summarized in table 2-1) there are some important exclusions from it. For example, the costs of medical and nursing education are excluded insofar as possible, and these form part of educational expenditures. The costs of administering the health-insurance plan are excluded, but costs of the Ministry of Health are included, as are hospital-administration costs. Some doctors are employed by private industry in connection with occupational-health programs, and their costs are not known to government and are not included in the health-expenditure calculations. Ambulance costs are included, but not the costs incurred by individuals in traveling by other forms of transport (154 million Kronor in 1974 and 204 million in 1975 are known to have been reclaimed from the health-insurance plan for this purpose—to include them would distort the comparisons with most other countries. If included, they would raise recorded total expenditure by less than 1 percent). As elsewhere, the boundary between health and welfare programs is arbitrary. In Sweden social-welfare institutions and programs are run by local government, whereas hospitals and medical programs are the responsibility of the county councils. The latter are included in health-care expenditures, whereas the former are not. This arrangement could exclude from health-care expenditures some services for the elderly and handicapped that would be included in, say, the Netherlands. On the other hand, the Swedish model of care is in general a medical one, so that medical services are broad in scope.

(6) *Government and private enterprise*: In Sweden virtually all hospitals are owned and administered by the government. Nonprofit, nongovernment hospitals are virtually unknown. The private, for-profit sector comprises principally the private practice of physicians, dentists, and nurses.

(7) *Care outside hospitals*: This item includes specialist care delivered on an ambulatory basis, as well as primary care. Costs of medicines prescribed on an ambulatory basis are also included.

(8) *Other services*: Expenditures on education for doctors and nurses are largely excluded (see note 5). Other educational costs, as well as the costs of public health programs, cannot be differentiated in the Swedish national accounts from the hospital and ambulatory-care headings (lines 13 and 15 in the tables).

(9) *Administration costs*: As stated in note 5, administrative costs of the insurance plan are not included. (The plan is, of course, primarily concerned with cash allowances, rather than with reimbursement of medical costs.) The costs of the Ministry of Health and of hospital administration should be included.

(10) *Manpower numbers*: The figures for manpower numbers are derived primarily from the National Board of Health and Welfare publication *Public Health in Sweden, 1975*, table B1. Unfortunately, this covers only the main health professions, plus hospital employees. Some auxiliary staff in hospitals, along with several categories of staff in physicians' offices and community clinics, are excluded. This helps to explain why the Central Bureau of Statistics' estimate for total health manpower (line 26) is substantially higher than the sum of the figures in the National Board's table B1. *However, both sets of figures make no adjustment for part-time workers.* Adjustments can be made on the following basis:

	Total Hours Worked	*Normal Working Time per Person*	*Whole-Time Equivalents*
1974	442,250,000	1690	261,700
1975	460,180,000	1690	272,300

This provides a manpower ratio (whole-time equivalent) per 10,000 population of 321 in 1974 and 332 in 1975. Both figures seem very high by comparison with the other countries included, the next highest figure being 218.6 for Switzerland. Accordingly, the Swedish figures have not been included in the summary ratios.

(11) *Equipment, supplies, and other*: Estimated as a residual, after deducting lines 26, 27, and 29 from total expenditure.

(12) *Buildings*: Derived from line 14 of the table and therefore covering hospital capital expenditure only. Most private expenditure on buildings (for example, on physicians' offices) is recovered through fees, rather than being identified as capital expenditure.

Table C-8
Switzerland
(millions of Swiss francs, unless stated otherwise)

	1974	1974 Percentage	1975	1975 Percentage	Notes
Basic data					
1. Population (thousands)	6,442.8		6,405.0		
2. GNP	146,495		144,390		
GDP	141,400		139,920		(1)
3. GNP per capita (francs)	22,738		22,543		
GDP per capita (francs)	21,947		21,845		
Health expenditure by source of finance					
4. Public					
(a) General taxation			3,128	31.6	(2)
(b) Public insurance			3,451	34.9	
			6,579	66.5	
5. Consumers					
(a) Private insurance			3,321	33.5	(2)
(b) Direct payment					
6. Other			—	—	
7. Total expenditure					
(a) Total			9,900	100.0	(3)
(b) Per capita (francs)			1,546		
(c) Percentage of GNP			6.86		
(d) Percentage of GDP			7.08		
Health expenditure by ownership/administration of channel of provision					
8. Government institutions (state-owned and -run)			3,778	38.1	
9. Nongovernment, not for profit			1,443	14.6	(4)
10. Private, for-profit institutions and contractors			4,679	47.3	
11. Other			—	—	
12. Total (8-11)			9,900	100.0	
Health expenditure by service					
13. Hospitals (current)			3,750	37.9	(5)
14. Hospitals (capital)			694	7.0	
			4,444	44.9	
15. Care outside hospitals					
(a) Primary care			4,055	41.0	(6)
(b) Specialist care					
(c) Capital expenditure					
16. Self-medication			500	5.0	

Table C-8 *(continued)*

	1974	1974 Percentage	1975	1975 Percentage	Notes
17. Other services					
(a) Public health			381	3.8	(7)
(b) Research			} 520	5.3	(8)
(c) Education					
(d) Other			—		
			901	9.1	
18. Administration			NA	—	(9)
19. Other			—	—	
20. Total (13-19)			9,900	100.0	

Health expenditure by resource

	Cost	Percentage	Number	Cost	Percentage	Number
Manpower						
21. Doctors						
(a) General practice						2,363
(b) All other						9,540
Dentists						
(a) General practice						3,900
(b) All other						
22. Nurses (qualified)						
23. Nurses (other) Total nursing						Approx. 124,000
24. Professional and technical						
25. Administrative and clerical and auxiliary						
26. Total manpower				6,395	64.6	Approx. 140,000
27. Pharmaceuticals						
(a) Prescribed				} 838	8.5	
(b) OTC drugs						
28. Equipment and supplies				1,973	19.9	
29. Buildings				694	7.0	
30. Other				—	—	
31. Total (21-30)				9,900	100.0	

Notes in right columns: 21. (10); 26. (11); 28. (13); 29. (12).

Source: The Swiss figures are based on Pierre Gygi and Heiner Henny, *Le système suisse de santé: dépenses, structure et formation des prix dans le domaine des soins médicaux,* (Bern: Hans Huber, 1977) 2d ed. See also P. Gygi, *"L'assurance—maladie en suisse,"* Les cahiers médico-sociaux (1978):39-45. I am most grateful to Pierre Gygi for his help in extracting and interpreting the figures. No comparable figures are available for 1974. References are to the numbers in the right-hand column of the Swiss tables.

NA = not available.

Reference notes:

(1) *Population, GNP, and so on:* The source of these figures is the *Statistical Yearbook* for Switzerland.

(2) *Sources of finance:* The makeup of the general-tax-public-insurance figures is as follows:

Table C-8 *(continued)*

	Millions of Swiss Francs	Percentage of Total Health-Care Expenditure
Direct and indirect taxation		
Federal	148	1.5
Cantons	2,610	26.4
Communes	370	3.7
	3,128	31.6
Publicly subsidized insurance		
Caisses-maladie	3,075	31.1
AM, AI, and CNA	376	3.8
	3,451	34.9

Subsidies from government to these insurance funds total approximately 1,000 million Swiss francs. Taking the subsidies into account raises the general-tax element to 41.7 percent and reduces the insurance element to 24.8 percent. (These adjusted percentages are the ones used in table 4-1.)

(3) *Total expenditure*: As in other countries, the boundary between health-care and other social expenditure depends on the classification of the administering agency, institution, or professional group concerned. Thus, finance for homes for the handicapped or the elderly, when not administered by a medical agency, is excluded except for payments to visiting physicians. Payments for home visits are included for doctors and nurses, but excluded for domestic help. Educational costs are included for clinical-training programs run by universities and hospitals, but excluded for private establishments, for example, those for training physicians' aides. Compared to the other countries surveyed, the definitions of health-care expenditure in Switzerland seem on the narrow side. The most obvious example of this is the general exclusion of transportation costs, even in the case of ambulances and medical helicopters. A second, less-precise example is administration: Government-administration costs are excluded (government playing a relatively small role in the Swiss health system except at the cantonal level), and the administration costs of the insurance companies are only partially included. As Gygi and Henny emphasize in *Le système suisse*, the Swiss figures are taken from many different sources because of the very decentralized nature of the government and the health-care system. These authors previously prepared a detailed analysis for 1973, and Pierre Gygi and Peter Tschopp had done so for 1965 in *Sécurité médico-sociale* (Bern, Hans Huber, 1968). Each time, in retrospect the analysis proved incomplete. Overall, Swiss health-care expenditures are probably somewhat understated relative to others, perhaps (as suggested in table 2-1) by an order of magnitude of 5-10 percent.

(4) *Ownership/administration*: The makeup is as follows:

	Millions of Swiss Francs	Percentage of Total Health-Care Expenditure
Public Institutions		
Public hospitals (40,000 beds)		
Current	2,143	21.6
Capital	694	7.0
Dental clinics	40	0.4
Public-health programs	381	3.8
University medical schools	520	5.3
	3,778	38.1
Private institutions delivering public services		
Hospitals (25,000 beds)	1,339	13.5
Domiciliary and other services	104	1.1
	1,443	14.6
Private, for-profit, including private practice		
Private hospitals (5,000 beds)	268	2.7
Doctors (including attached pharmacies)	2,120	21.4
Medical laboratories	50	0.5

Table C-8 *(continued)*

Chiropractors	19	0.2
Physiotherapists	45	0.5
Dentists	905	9.1
Pharmacies	822	8.3
Chemists (pharmaceutical specialties only)	150	1.5
Miscellaneous providers	300	3.1
	4,679	47.3

(5) *Hospital costs (current)*: Amortization for periods under three years *is* included in running costs.

(6) *Care outside hospital*: These figures represent the cost of ambulatory treatment and of treatment in the home under medical supervision. They include:

	Millions of Swiss Francs	Percentage of Total Health-Care Expenditure
Doctors (including attached pharmacies)	2,120	21.4
Medical laboratories	50	0.5
Chiropractors	19	0.2
Physiotherapists	45	0.5
Dentists	945	9.5
Domiciliary and other services	104	1.1
Pharmacies	472	4.8
Miscellaneous providers	300	3.0
	4,055	41.0

(7) *Public health*: Public-health services include the campaigns against tuberculosis and polio, the campaign against alcoholism, control of food products, administration, and so on.

(8) *Research and education*: These represent the costs of university medical schools. Some other research and education costs are no doubt included in hospital costs (line 13). Education costs in private establishments (for example, training of physicians' aides) are excluded. Research by pharmaceutical companies is excluded here but included in the costs of pharmaceutical products. There are no major medical-research centers or foundations in Switzerland other than those in hospitals, universities, and the pharmaceutical companies.

(9) *Administration costs*: Costs of administration are not separately available. In part they are included elsewhere (for example, lines 13 and 17a) and in part they are excluded from this analysis (see note 3).

(10) *Doctors and dentists*: See Gygi and Henny, *Le système suisse* p. 53, table 10, and p. 83.

(11) *Total manpower*: See Gygi, *L'assurance maladie en suisse*, pp. 40, 45.

(12) *Buildings*: Hospital capital expenditure only is included here (see line 14) since that is the only capital expenditure that can be separately identified. It is charged when incurred for major projects. Relatively minor expenditure can be amortized over a period of up to three years and is then included in current costs. Capital expenditure in the private sector (for example, that of private practitioners) is recovered through market price and is included in line 28.

(13) *Equipment and supplies*: This line is derived as a residual and includes capital expenditure outside hospitals.

Table C-9
United Kingdom
(millions of pounds sterling, unless stated otherwise)

| | 1974-1975 | | | | |
| | England | | United Kingdom | | |
	Cost	Percentage	Cost	Percentage	Notes
Basic data					
1. Population (thousands)	46,400		55,922		(1)
2. GNP			83,478		
GDP			82,196		(2)
3. GNP per capita (pounds)			1,493		
GDP per capita (pounds)			1,470		
Health expenditure by source of finance					
4. Public					
(a) General taxation	3,264	86.7	4,051	87.3	
(b) Compulsory insurance	197	5.2	(232)	5.0	(3)
(c) Other	14	0.4	(16)	0.3	
	3,475	92.3	4,299	92.6	
5. Consumers					
(a) Voluntary insurance	(47)	1.3	55	1.2	(4)
(b) Direct payment	223	5.9	267	5.8	(5)
	270	7.2	322	7.0	
6. Other	18	0.5	20	0.4	(6)
7. Total expenditure					
(a) Total	3,763	100.0	4,641	100.0	(7)
(b) Per capita (pounds)	81.1		83.0		
(c) Percentage of GNP	(5.01)		5.24		(2)
(d) Percentage of GDP	(5.08)		5.31		
Health expenditure by ownership/administration of channel of provision					
8. Government institutions (state-owned and -run)	2,833	75.3	3,401	73.3	
9. Nongovernment, not for profit	Negligible	—	Negligible	—	(8)
10. Private, for-profit institutions and contractors	930	24.7	1,240	26.7	
11. Other	—	—	—	—	
12. Total (8-11)	3,763	100.0	4,641	100.0	
Health expenditure by service					
13. Hospitals (current)	2,153	57.2	2,640	56.9	(9)
14. Hospitals (capital)	247	6.6	273	5.9	(10)
	2,400	63.8	2,913	62.8	
15. Care outside hospitals					
(a) Primary care	706	18.8	967	20.8	(11)
(b) Specialist care	—		—		
(c) Capital expenditure	20	0.5	24	0.5	(10)
16. Self-medication	(128)	3.4	150	3.2	(12)

Table C-9 *(continued)*

	England		United Kingdom		
		1974-1975			
	Cost	Percentage	Cost	Percentage	Notes
17. Other services					
(a) Public health	244	6.5	286	6.2	(13)
(b) Research	68	1.8	72	1.5	(14)
(c) Education	—	—	—	—	(15)
18. Administration	34	0.9	(39)	0.9	(16)
19. Other	163	4.3	190	4.1	(17)
20. Total (13-19)	3,763	100.0	4,641	100.0	

	Cost	Per-centage	Number (thousands) Whole Time Equiva-lents	Cost	Per-centage	Number (thousands) Whole Time Equiva-lents
Health expenditure by resource						
Manpower						
21. Doctors						
(a) General practice	200	5.3	21			
(b) All other	220	5.9	32			
	420	11.2	53			
Dentists						
(a) General practice	72	1.9	11			
(b) All other	11	.3	4			
	83	2.2	15			
22. Nurses (qualified)	464	12.3	124			
23. Nurses (other)	297	7.9	208			(18)
Total nursing	761	20.2	332			
24. Professional and technical	220	5.8	95			
25. Administrative and clerical and auxiliary	691	18.4	257			
26. Total manpower	2,176	57.8	752			

	Cost	Percent		Cost	Percent	
27. Pharmaceuticals						
(a) Prescribed	351	9.3		(413)	8.9	(19)
(b) OTC drugs	(128)	3.4		150	3.2	
	479	12.7		563	12.1	
28. Equipment and supplies	577	15.4				(20)
29. Buildings	267	7.1		307	6.6	
30. Other	264	7.0		300	6.5	(21)
31. Total (21-30)	3,763	100.0		4,641	100.0	

Table C-9
United Kingdom
(millions of pounds sterling 1975-1978, unless stated otherwise)

	England		United Kingdom		
	Cost	Percentage	Cost	Percentage	Notes
Basic data					
1. Population (thousands)	46,391		55,900.5		(1)
2. GNP per capita			103,692		
GDP per capita			102,929		(2)
3. GNP per capita (pounds)			1,855		
GDP per capita (pounds)			1,841		
Health expenditure by source of finance					
4. Public					
(a) General taxation	4,139	84.7	5,158	85.5	
(b) Compulsory insurance	398	8.1	(471)	7.8	(3)
(c) Other	14	0.3	(16)	0.3	
	4,551	93.1	5,645	93.6	
5. Consumers					
(a) Voluntary insurance	(60)	1.2	71	1.2	(4)
(b) Direct payment	257	5.3	295	4.9	(5)
	317	6.5	366	6.1	
6. Other	20	0.4	22	0.4	(6)
7. Total expenditure					
(a) Total	4,888	100.0	6,033	100.0	(7)
(b) Per capita (pounds)	105.4		107.9		
(c) Percentage of GNP	(5.32)		5.55		(2)
(d) Percentage of GDP	(5.36)		5.59		
Health expenditure by ownership/administration of channel of provision					
8. Government institutions (state-owned and -run)	3,702	75.7	4,579	75.9	
9. Nongovernment, not for profit	Negligible	—	Negligible	—	(8)
10. Private, for-profit institutions and contractors	1,186	24.3	1,454	24.1	
11. Other	—	—	—	—	
12. Total (8-11)	4,888	100.0	6,033	100.0	
Health expenditure by service					
13. Hospitals (current)	2,818	57.7	3,634	60.2	(9)
14. Hospitals (capital)	307	6.2	326	5.4	(10)
	3,125	63.9	3,960	65.6	
15. Care outside hospitals					
(a) Primary care	939	19.2	1,141	18.9	(11)
(b) Specialist care	—		—		
(c) Capital expenditure	25	0.5	(29)	0.5	(10)
16. Self-medication	(153)	3.1	180	3.0	(12)

Table C-9 *(continued)*

	England		United Kingdom		Notes
	1975-1976				
	Cost	*Percentage*	*Cost*	*Percentage*	
17. Other services					
(a) Public health	323	6.6	381	6.3	(13)
(b) Research	80	1.6	86	1.4	(14)
(c) Education	—	—	—	—	(15)
18. Administration	45	0.9	53	0.9	(16)
19. Other	198	4.2	203	3.4	(17)
20. Total (13-19)	4,888	100.0	6,033	100.0	
	Cost	*Number*	*Cost*	*Number*	

Health expenditure by resource

Manpower

21. Doctors				
(a) General practice				
(b) All other				
Dentists				
(a) General practice				
(b) All other				
22. Nurses (qualified)	See 1974-1975 for			
23. Nurses (other)	breakdown for England			
Total nursing				
24. Professional and technical				
25. Administrative and clerical and auxiliary				
26. Total manpower				
	Cost	*Percent*	*Cost*	*Percent*
27. Pharmaceuticals				
(a) Prescribed				
(b) OTC drugs	(153)	3.1	180	3.0
28. Equipment and supplies				
29. Buildings	332	6.8	367	6.1
30. Other				
31. Total (21-30)	4,888	100.0	6,033	100.0

Source: The sources of the U.K. figures, which are primarily various U.K. government statistical publications, are given in the notes that follow. References are to the numbers in the right-hand column of the statistical tables for the United Kingdom. A peculiarity of all British data is the use of different national entities for different statistics, without regard for analysts who might be trying to relate one set of data to another. Some figures are given for the United Kingdom, some for Great Britain (that is, the United Kingdom, excluding Northern Ireland), some for England and Wales, and some for England only. For no one of these national entities are all the figures complete. I have therefore compiled each year's figures in two columns, one for the United Kingdom and the other for England, estimating one column from the other when necessary. In using the tables as the source for international comparisons in this book, I have taken the U.K. column, including the estimates that it contains, except for the manpower numbers and resource breakdown, for which I have had to use the ratios for England. Concerning dates, I have calculated expenditures on the basis of fiscal years to 31 March, because these are the periods for which National Health Service (NHS) expenditures are published.

Table C-9 *(continued)*

Reference notes:

(1) *Population*: Mid-calendar-year estimates from the Central Office of Information.

(2) *GNP/GDP*: GNP and GDP for the United Kingdom are from *National Income and Expenditure 1967-77*, Central Statistical Office, table 1.1 They are at market prices for calendar years. GNP is not calculated for England on its own, and GDP is given in the regional statistics for England only at factor cost. Where (as noted in the tables by a figure in brackets) I have used the ratio (U.K. GDP at factor cost)/(England GDP at factor cost) to estimate a missing statistic, I have taken both figures from the regional statistics, for consistency. To calculate health-care expenditures as a percentage of GNP and GDP (lines 7c and d), I have estimated fiscal-year GNP and GDP (to 31 March) by taking 75 percent of the preceding calendar year and 25 percent of the current calendar year.

(3) *Public finance*: The National Health Service is financed primarily by direct payments from the central government's Consolidated Fund (line 4a), with subsidiary funding from compulsory contributions (see line 4b) and charges for certain services (included in line 5b). The main source of the data for England is the Department of Health and Social Security (DHSS) Annual Reports for 1975 and 1976, and for the United Kingdom is *Social Trends*, no. 7 (1976):149, table 2.30. The *Social Trends* figures are not set out in exactly the same way. Total public expenditure on health care in the United Kingdom is calculated as follows:

		1974-1975 *Millions of* *Pounds*		1975-1976 *Millions of* *Pounds*
Total public expenditure on health and personal social services, as given in *Social Trends*		5,325 –		7,022 –
Less:				
Personal social services (current)	739		999	
School milk	9		13	
School meals (net of charges)	304		399	
Personal social services (capital)	83		91	
		1,135		1,502
		4,190		5,520
Plus:				
Medical services for the armed forces		78		85
Government research expenditure from sources other than the DHSS		31		40
		4,299		5,645

(4) *Voluntary insurance*: Subscription income for the United Kingdom from *UK Private Medical Care 1977* by Lee Donaldson Associates. The figure for England is estimated from the U.K. figure. I have not tried to adjust Donaldson's calendar-year figure to a fiscal-year basis.

(5) *Direct payment*: This line comprises NHS charges for services, expenditure on over-the-counter drugs (see line 27b) and Donaldson's estimate of patients' payments for health services, less benefits. Donaldson's estimate of patients' payments is for U.K. residents registered with the three largest schemes, accounting for 98 percent of all subscriptions. It thus excludes payments by foreigners coming to the United Kingdom for treatment. It also excludes items that would not fall within the NHS definition of health care, such as osteopathy, cosmetic surgery, and health farms. Finally, Donaldson's estimate excludes direct payment by U.K. residents who are not registered with any insurance scheme.

(6) *Other*: This item represents funding from charities for medical research.

(7) *Total expenditure*: The total includes the cost of the National Health Service and of medical services for the armed forces, and estimated costs for private medical care and for nonprescribed drugs. There can be little argument about the accuracy of NHS expenditures, which make up some 90 percent of the total. The private sector could be underestimated, but the estimate is based on the best source available; moreover, even a substantial revision would make little difference to total expenditures. As in most other countries surveyed, the costs of university education are excluded. Clinical education and training are included. Research expenditure covers spending by the Medical Research Council, the Department of Health (and to a minor extent other government departments), and charities. Research expenditure by pharmaceutical and supply companies is included in prices paid for these products. Most administrative costs are included, although the major part of these is included in the costs of hospital and other services; central-government costs are included, as is the difference between the income of insurance companies and benefits paid. Ambulance costs are included, but traveling costs met privately by individuals are excluded. For public-health and environmental services only the costs of medical supervision are included. As in other countries, the boundary between health and social-welfare expenditure depends on who runs the service, under what government vote it is financed, and whether there is medical supervision. By U.K. definitions the personal social services include residential homes (not under medical supervision) for the elderly and physically handicapped, a substantial range of home-care and day-center activities, children's homes, and social work for

Table C-9 *(continued)*

individuals and families. Accordingly, these are excluded from health-care expenditures. Overall, the U.K. figures appear to be comprehensive.

(8) *Expenditure by ownership/administration*: The government sector comprises the following for 1974-1975:

	England Millions of Pounds	United Kingdom Millions of Pounds
Health authorities (current)	2,351	2,872
Health authorities (capital)	267	297
Welfare foods	8	9
Central administration	25 ⎫	163
Other	116 ⎭	
	2,767	3,323
Medical services for the armed forces	(66)	78
	2,833	3,401

The calculation for 1975-1976 is parallel. The general medical, dental, and ophthalmic services are excluded from the government sector since they are delivered by independent practitioners on the basis of contracts for services.

(9) *Hospital expenditure (current)*: This line is estimated as follows for 1974-1975:

	England Millions of Pounds	United Kingdom Millions of Pounds
Current spending by health authorities	2,351 −	2,872 −
Less: Estimated expenditure on community-health services at the 1973-1974 figure of 5.75 percent of total public spending on health and personal social services	236	(277)
	2,115 +	2,595 +
Plus: All inpatient charges paid by private patients (BUPA, PPP, WPA)	(38)	45
	2,153	2,640

The calculation for 1975-1976 is done on the same basis.

(10) *Hospital expenditure (capital)*: Line 14 represents capital expenditure by health authorities, less an estimate of expenditure on health centers and other community-health facilities (line 15c). The latter is derived from information for England in the Department of Health Annual Report, 1976, p. 36, table 14. Capital expenditure by the private sector is not included but has been minute until very recently.

(11) *Primary care*: This includes the following for 1974-1975:

	England Millions of Pounds	United Kingdom Millions of Pounds
General medical services	211	
Pharmaceutical services	300	
General dental services	153	
General ophthalmic services	36	
	700	960
Plus private payment for outpatient care	6	7
	706	967

The same method of calculation was used for 1975-1976.

Table C-9 *(continued)*

(12) *Self-medication*: The source for this figure for the United Kingdom is the Office of Health Economics. I have taken their estimate of sales at consumer prices. Their figures were on a calendar-year basis and have been adjusted slightly to bring them into line with fiscal years.

(13) *Public health*: Expenditure on public-health activities, such as health inspection, disease control, and child-health clinics, has not been separately recorded since the NHS reorganization of 1974. The estimate is derived from the ratio of local-authority health services to total health and personal social-services expenditure in England in 1973-1974 (see note 9). To this I have added expenditure on welfare foods.

(14) *Research*: I estimate research expenditure for the United Kingdom as follows:

	1974-1975 Millions of Pounds	1975-1976 Millions of Pounds	1976-1977 Millions of Pounds
Medical Research Council (MRC)	36.3	46.6	52.2
DHSS (net of transfers to the MRC)	13.5	15.1	15.8
Other government expenditure on medical research	2.2	2.3	2.5
	52.0	64.0	70.5
Charities	20.0	22.0	25.0
Total	72.0	86.0	95.5

The England estimate is derived from this. In neither case is research expenditure by industry included, on the grounds that this would involve double counting.

(15) *Education*: Preclinical education costs for doctors, and the costs of educating science and other graduates, are excluded. In-service training costs are included, particularly in line 13, but are not separately identifiable.

(16) *Administration*: Included here are the cost of central administration, as well as subscription income less benefits paid under voluntary insurance schemes. The 1974-1975 calculation is:

	England Millions of Pounds		United Kingdom Millions of Pounds
Central administration	25		(30)
Subscription income		55	
Less benefits		46	
	(9)		9
	34		39

Other costs of administration, particularly those of the health authorities, are included in line 13 and elsewhere. For the NHS as a whole, a review of administration was carried out in 1976 with the aim of cutting total administrative costs from 5.7 percent of the budget to 5.25 percent.

(17) *Other*: This line comprises for England other costs of the health and personal social services, as shown in the DHSS annual report, less expenditure on research, plus expenditure on medical services for the armed forces. The calculation for the United Kingdom is similar, using the data in *Social Trends*, except that an allowance must also be made for central administration, which is not separately identified in *Social Trends*.

(18) *Manpower numbers and costs*: Manpower numbers for England are derived from *Health and Personal Social Services Statistics for England, 1977*, tables 3.2 and (for details of nursing staff) 3.15. They are mainly in the form of whole-time equivalents, although family practitioners and their staff, representing roughly 5 percent of the total, are not adjusted for part-time working. Manpower costs were derived, with the help of J.W. Hurst of the Department of Health, from the subjective analysis of revenue expenditure for hospital and community-health services, with information from the annual accounts of the Family Practitioner Services. To the cost of doctors I have added £ 20 million for fees paid for private medical care, representing the nonaccommodation element of Donaldson's estimate for the United Kingdom, in 1975, adjusted to an estimate for England. I have not been able to obtain a breakdown by resource of medical expenditure for the various items included in line 30, such as medical expenditure for the armed forces and research expenditure. If, as seems highly probable, these all contain a similar manpower element to the bulk of health expenditure, then salaries and wages increase as a proportion of total expenditure from the 57.8 percent shown on line 26 to 62 percent.

(19) *Pharmaceuticals*: The costs of pharmaceuticals are estimated as follows, for England in 1974-1975:

Table C-9 *(continued)*

	Millions of Pounds
Pharmaceutical services (from DHSS Annual Report)	300
Hospital drugs (from the subjective analysis of revenue expenditure)	51
Total prescribed	351
OTC drugs (from line 16)	128
	479

(20) *Equipment and supplies*: This figure is derived as a residual.

(21) *Other*: Included here are various items for which I have been unable to obtain a resource breakdown, namely for 1974-1975:

	England Millions of Pounds	United Kingdom Millions of Pounds
Research expenditure	68	72
Other services (line 19)	163	190
Private medical care (less fees included in line 21)		
Payments by patients for accommodation	(25)	29
Difference between subscription income and benefits	8	9
	264	300

Table C-10
United States
(millions of dollars, unless stated otherwise)

	1974-1975	1974-1975 Percentage	1975-1976	1975-1976 Percentage	Notes (1)
Basic data					
1. Population (thousands)	217,031		218,843		(2)
2. GNP	1,487,100		1,667,400		
3. GNP per capita (dollars)	6,852.0		7,617.3		(3)
Health expenditure by source of finance					
4. Public					
(a) General taxation	(39,532)	(31.0)	(44,310)	(30.5)	(4)
(b) Public insurance	(14,948)	(11.7)	(17,232)	(11.9)	
	54,481	42.7	61,542	42.4	
5. Consumers					
(a) Private insurance	28,514	22.3	33,618	23.1	(5)
(b) Direct payment	34,697	27.1	39,425	27.2	
(c) Other	4,164	3.3	4,427	3.1	(6)
	67,375	52.7	77,470	53.4	
6. Other	5,862	4.6	6,090	4.2	(7)
7. Total expenditure					
(a) Total	127,719	100.0	145,102	100.0	
(b) Per capita (dollars)	588.5		663.1		
(c) Percentage of GNP	8.6		8.7		
(d) Percentage of GDP	—		—		
Health expenditure by ownership/administration of channel of provision					
8. Government institutions (state-owned and -run)	24,330	19.0	26,926	18.6	
9. Nongovernment, not for profit					
	103,389	81.0	118,176	81.4	(9)
10. Private, for-profit institutions and contractors					
11. Other	—		—		
12. Total (8-11)	127,719	100.0	145,102	100.0	
Health expenditure by service					
13. Hospitals (current)	49,973	39.1	57,497	39.6	(10)
14. Hospitals (capital)	4,815	3.8	5,111	3.5	(11)
	54,788	42.9	62,608	43.1	
15. Care outside hospitals					
(a) Primary care					
(b) Specialist care					
(c) Capital expenditure	51,072	40.0	57,887	39.9	(12)
16. Self-medication					

Table C-10 *(continued)*

	1974-1975	1974-1975 Percentage	1975-1976	1975-1976 Percentage	Notes (1)
17. Other services					
(a) Public health	3,091	2.4	3,522	2.4	(13)
(b) Research	3,132	2.5	3,623	2.5	
(c) Education	Excluded		Excluded		
18. Administration	6,016	4.7	6,628	4.6	(14)
19. Other—nursing home care	9,620	7.5	10,834	7.5	
20. Total (13-19)	127,719	100.0	145,102	100.0	

	Cost	Number	Cost	Number

Health expenditure by resource

Manpower

	1974-1975	1974-1975	1975-1976	1975-1976	
21. Doctors					
(a) General practice		53,150		53,700	
(b) All other		295,750		310,800	
Total		348,900			
Dentists		100,000		110,000	
22. Nurses (qualified)		904,000		935,000	(15) and (16)
23. Nurses (other)		1,308,000		1,372,000	
Total nursing		2,212,000		2,307,000	
24. Professional and technical		1,312,100*		1,387,500*	
25. Administrative and clerical and auxiliary					
26. Total manpower		3,973,000*		4,169,000*	

	1974-1975	1974-1975 Percentage	1975-1976	1975-1976 Percentage	Notes (1)
27. Pharmaceuticals					
(a) Prescribed	10,582	8.3	11,472	7.9	(16)
(b) OTC drugs					
28. Equipment and supplies					
29. Buildings	4,815	3.8	5,111	3.5	
30. Other					
31. Total (21-30)	127,719	100.0	145,102	100.0	

Source: The source for the American figures is DHEW in Washington. Each year for some time, the figures have been published in exemplary fashion in the *Social Security Bulletin*; and there is an unparalleled series of health-care-expenditure statistics dating back to 1929. Unfortunately, the format differs from mine in several ways. For example, it contains no manpower costs or statistics. Therefore, I have had to estimate a number of figures (which are printed in brackets), and to leave some gaps. I am grateful to Robert Derzon, former head of the Health Care Financing Administration, and to Robert M. Gibson for their interest in the project. References are to the numbers in the right-hand column of the American tables.

Note: * = Incomplete (health occupations only).

Reference notes:

(1) *Dates*: The periods are fiscal years to 30 September (the U.S. federal government's fiscal year has recently changed from July through June, to October through September).

Table C-10 *(continued)*

(2) *Population*: For 1 April (mid-fiscal year), based on data from the Bureau of the Census. See R.M. Gibson and C.R. Fisher, *Social Security Bulletin* 41, no. 7 (July 1978):20.

(3) *GNP*: See Gibson and Fisher, *Social Security Bulletin*, table 1.

(4) *General taxation and public insurance*: Total public financing is given in Gibson and Fisher, *Social Security Bulletin*, but not the breakdown between general taxation and public insurance. This is estimated for 1974-1975 as follows, from tables 2 and 4 in the same article and from information about Medicare receipts on page 16:

		General Taxation Millions of Dollars		Public Insurance Millions of Dollars
Medicare	(16 percent)	2,633	(83.1 percent)	12,947
Disability insurance (medical benefits)				75
Workers compensation (medical benefits)				1,926
Medicaid		13,245		
Other public assistance		670		
General hospital and medical care		7,503		
Defense-department hospital and medical care		3,132		
Maternal- and child-health services		558		
Public-health activities		3,091		
Veterans' Administration		3,426		
Medical vocational rehabilitation		265		
Research and construction		5,009		
		39,532		14,948
			54,481	

The 1975-1976 estimate was done in exactly the same way.

(5) *Private insurance*: The figures in this line are for benefits paid under private health insurance, from Gibson and Fisher, *Social Security Bulletin*, table 3.

(6) *Consumers (other)*: Expenses for prepayment and administration under private insurance (premiums less benefits).

(7) *Other payers*: These include payments by philanthropic organizations and payments by employers for occupational health services.

(8) *Total expenditure*: The American definition of health expenditures embraces all medical care, medical research, health administration, and construction. *All expenditure for education and training of health professionals is excluded*, so that the American figures are in this respect understated compared with those for most of the other countries surveyed, which include clinical education and training. The boundary between health and welfare programs is in principle quite sharply drawn. All hospital expenditures are included, and hospitals must by definition have a medical staff. Nursing homes, in order to qualify as health institutions, must have at least half their residents receiving nursing care (this means, of course, that up to half can be elderly people requiring little medical or nursing care). Social-work assistance of any kind is classified as welfare, not health-care expenditure. Ambulance costs are included in health-care expenditures, but any other transport costs for patients are not. Administrative costs are comprehensive, covering the operation of all public programs (including an allocated share of DHEW's costs) and benefits less premiums for private health insurance; hospital administration is included in hospital costs. For environmental services, like water supply and sanitation, only medical supervision (the traditional public-health-service component) is included, not the basic costs of the services themselves. There is a small element of double counting in capital costs since expenditures are charged initially and by way of depreciation in subsequent years. Gibson and Fisher, in *Social Security Bulletin*, p. 19, state that this "duplication is estimated to be small, not significantly affecting total health expenditures." See table 2-1 for an overall assessment of comparability.

(9) *Ownership/administration*: This breakdown is not available from DHEW. I have estimated it very roughly from Gibson and Fisher, *Social Security Bulletin*, tables 2 and 4, on the following basis:

Table C-10 *(continued)*

Government Institutions	1974-1975 Millions of Dollars	1975-1976 Millions of Dollars
General hospital and medical care (Indian Health Service, and so on)	7,503	7,845
Defense department	3,132	3,203
Maternal- and child-health services	588	604
Public-health activities	3,091	3,522
Veterans' Administration	3,426	3,932
Medical vocational rehabilitation	265	278
Prepayment and administration	1,346	1,643
Research	2,854	3,348
Construction	2,155	2,551
	24,330	26,926
Percentage of total expenditure	19.0	18.6
Nongovernment percentage (by deduction)	81.0	81.4

This estimation is oversimplified since, for example, municipal-government hospitals receive some of the funding through Medicaid and Medicare rather than directly; conversely, some public expenditure on research and construction is no doubt for projects at nongovernment institutions. By analogy with other countries and from some knowledge of the U.S. system, the following can be atttributed with reasonable certainty to the for-profit sector:

	1974-1975 Millions of Dollars	1975-1976 Millions of Dollars
Private expenditures for personal health care, *excluding* hospital care	44,282	50,270
Public expenditures under Medicare, Medicaid, and so on for physicians', dentists', other professional services and for drugs, glasses, appliances, and nursing-home care	12,977	14,594
	57,259	64,864
Percentage of total expenditure	44.8	44.7

This would leave about 36 percent of total expenditures, primarily representing hospital expenditures and nongovernment administration, in doubt between for-profit and nonprofit.

(10) *Hospital expenditure (current)*: The DHEW figures are based on data collected by the American Hospital Association. *They exclude private physicians' fees charged to patients for hospital care*. These charges are instead included in line 15 and cannot be differentiated accurately. *Anesthesia and radiology are sometimes classified as hospital expenses and sometimes as expenditures for physicians' services, depending on billing practices*. Hospital operating costs include some depreciation charges, and, as noted previously, there is therefore some double counting in the totals. Note that DHEW classifies nursing-home costs (line 19) separately from hospital costs.

(11) *Capital costs*: Line 14 includes *all* construction of medical facilities, other than private-practice facilities. Thus part of the expenditure properly relates to care outside hospitals.

(12) *Care outside hospitals*: This item includes the following from table 2 of Gibson and Fisher, *Social Security Bulletin*:

	1974-1975 Millions of Dollars	1975-1976 Millions of Dollars
Physicians' services	24,553	28,504
Dentists' services	8,034	8,987
Other professional services	2,463	2,849
Drugs and drug sundries	10,582	11,472
Glasses and appliances	1,822	1,986
Other health services	3,616	4,088
Rounding	2	1
	51,072	57,887

Table C-10 *(continued)*

Other health services include occupational-health services provided by employers, school health services, federal medical activities outside hospitals, and residual items.

(13) *Other services*: See Gibson and Fisher, *Social Security Bulletin*, table 2, and notes on definitions. Public health includes all federal outlays for the prevention and control of health problems, as well as conventional public-health activities by the states and local health departments, but not basic environmental services like sanitation and water supplies. Research includes all public and private medical research, except that of drug and medical-supply companies, which are recovered through the cost of the product. Unlike those for the other countries surveyed, which generally include some education and training costs, the DHEW analysis seeks to exclude them all.

(14) *Administration*: These expenses comprise the administrative costs (where they are separately identified) of all federally financed health programs, and premiums less benefits for private health-insurance organizations. Hospital-administration expenses are included in hospital costs, and the same is true for ambulatory and nursing-home care.

(15) *Manpower numbers*: Manpower numbers for 1974 and 1975 are from *Health United States, 1979*, (Washington, 1979) published by DHEW, pp. 212, 213, tables 48, 49. Table 49 has been used for professionally active physicians (excluding osteopaths), since it seems comparable with WHO figures. Table 48 has been used for all other manpower numbers, recognizing that the figures are for *health-related occupations only* and thus exclude large groups of ancillary personnel like hospital cleaners and catering staff. Table 47 in *Health United States, 1979* gives census figures for those employed in the health-service industry. The totals are 5,554,000 for 1974 and 5,865,000 for 1975. The resulting ratios per 10,000 population (256 in 1974 and 268 in 1975) are very high by international standards and presumably include many part-time workers. They have not been used for purposes of comparisons.

(16) *Health expenditure by resource category*: It is surprising that DHEW health-care expenditure statistics give so little information by resource category. Nor does it seem possible to obtain reliable information from any other source, particularly for services other than hospital services. Expenditure on medical-facilities construction is available from DHEW. *Expenditure on drugs and drug sundries exclude drugs prescribed for hospital and nursing-home inpatients, and through physicians' offices*. It is therefore an underestimate of the total, even though it includes payment for some items that are not, strictly speaking, drugs. I have been unable to obtain any more comprehensive estimate from other sources. No information is available from DHEW on equipment and supplies expenditure, other than the relatively small item, glasses and appliances (see note 12), which again excludes hospital equipment and supplies. Information is totally absent on manpower costs, despite their crucial importance. Using information from *Trends Affecting the U.S. Health Care System*, DHEW (January 1976), exhibit IV-26 one can deduce that net annual earnings (after expenses) of U.S. physicians in 1972 were on the order of $50,000. Accepting this figure and applying it to the number of active physicians in that year (332,000) gives a total net-earnings figure of $16,600,000 or 17.9 percent of national health expenditures in the same period. This percentage is similar to that for Canada (17.9), France (17.3), and the Netherlands (17.0).

Appendix D:
Bibliographical
References

1. See the annual series of U.S. health-care expenditures regularly in the *Social Security Bulletin* by Department of Health, Education, and Welfare (DHEW) staff, for example, R.M. Gibson and C.R. Fisher, *Social Security Bulletin* 41, no. 7 (July 1978). The latest published figures (for 1979) appeared in an article by R.M. Gibson in *Health Care Financing Review*, Summer 1980.
2. See, for example, *La Dépense Nationale de Santé en 1977* and *La Consommation Médicale Finale 1979, Evaluations Provisoires.* Also see such publications as *La Pharmacie dans le Système de Santé Suède/France* (1977), *Comparaison des Dépenses de Santé en France et aux U.S.A. 1950-1978,* and *Analyse Régionale des Relations entre L'Offre et la Consommation de Soins Médicaux (secteur privé)* (1977). All published by CREDOC, Paris.
3. See *National Health Expenditures in Canada 1960-1975* (Ottawa: Health and Welfare Canada, 1979).
4. *International Labor Office, The Cost of Medical Care* (Geneva: ILO, 1959).
5. B. Abel-Smith, *Paying for Health Services,* Public Health Papers, no. 17 (Geneva: World Health Organization [WHO], 1963).
6. B. Abel-Smith, *An International Study of Health Expenditure,* Public Health Papers, no. 32 (Geneva: WHO, 1967).
7. J.G. Simanis, "International Health Expenditures," *Social Security Bulletin,* December 1970; and "Medical Care Expenditures in Seven Countries," *Social Security Bulletin,* March 1973.
8. *Public Expenditure on Health,* OECD Studies in Resource Allocation, no. 4 (Paris: Organization for Economic Cooperation and Development [OECD], July 1977).
9. B. Abel-Smith and A. Maynard, *The Organisation, Financing and Cost of Health Care in the European Community* (Brussels: European Economic Community [EEC], 1978).
10. B. Abel-Smith and P. Grandjeat, *Pharmaceutical Consumption* (Brussels: EEC, 1978).
11. H. Hauser and K. Koch, *Health Care Expenditure and its Financing— An International Survey,* mimeographed, 1979.
12. M.H. Cooper and A.J. Cooper, *International Price Comparison* (London: National Economic Development Office [NEDO], 1972); and M.H. Cooper, *European Pharmaceutical Prices, 1964-74* (London: Croom Helm, 1975).

13. Sir Derrick Dunlop and R.S. Inch, "Variations in Pharmaceutical and Medical Practice in Europe," *British Medical Journal*, 23 September 1972, pp. 749-752.

14. See, for example, the study by CREDOC *La Pharmacie dans le Système de Santé Suède/France* [2] and Abel-Smith and Grandjeat, *Pharmaceutical Consumption* [10].

15. W.A. Glaser, *Paying the Doctor* (Baltimore, Md.: Johns Hopkins Press, 1970).

16. W.A. Glaser, *Health Insurance Bargaining: Foreign Lessons for America* (New York: Gardner Press, 1978).

17. J.P. Bunker, "Surgical Manpower: A Comparison of Operations and Surgeons in the United States and in England and Wales, *New England Journal of Medicine 282* (1977):135; R. Kohn and Kerr L. White, *Health Care: An International Study* (London: Oxford University Press, Oxford Medical Publications, 1976); R.J.C. Pearson et al., "Hospital Case Loads in Liverpool, New England and Uppsala," *Lancet*, 7 September 1968; and Kerr L. White and J.H. Murnaghan, *International Comparison of Medical Care Utilization: A Feasibility Study* (Washington, D.C.: National Center for Health Statistics, 1969).

18. Descriptive work for groups of countries includes the following: O.W. Anderson, *Health Care: Can There be Equity?* (New York: Wiley, 1972); J. Blanpain, *National Health Insurance and Health Resources* (Cambridge, Mass.,: Harvard University Press, 1978); J. Bryant, *Health and the Developing World* (Ithaca, N.Y.: Cornell University Press, 1969); J. Douglas-Wilson and G. McLachlan, eds., *Health Services Prospects: An International Survey* (London: Lancet and Nuffield Provincial Hospitals Trust, 1973); J. Fry and W.J. Farndale, eds., *International Medical Care* (Oxford and Lancaster: Medical and Technical Publishing Co., 1972); M. Kaser, *Health Care in the Soviet Union and Eastern Europe* (London: Croom Helm, 1976); P.W. Kent, ed., *International Aspects of the Provision of Medical Care* (London and Boston, Mass.: Oriel Press, 1976); A. Maynard, *Health Care in the European Community* (London: Croom Helm, 1975); M. Ryan, *The Organisation of Soviet Medical Care* (Oxford and London: Basil Blackwell, and Martin Robertson, 1978); and J.G. Simanis, *National Health Systems in Eight Countries* (Washington, D.C.: DHEW, 1975).

19. For bibliographies on health economics, see: A.J. Culyer, J. Wiseman, and A. Walker, *An Annotated Bibliography of Health Economics* (London: Martin Robertson, 1977); and J.G. Cullis and P.A. West, *The Economics of Health: An Introduction* (London: Martin Robertson, 1979). For a more personal account of the evolution of thinking in health economics, see: H.E. Klarman, "Health Economics and Health Economics Research," *Millbank Memorial Fund Quarterly 57*, no. 3

(1979). Among the books that I personally have found most helpful on health economics in the broader context of social policy are: M.H. Cooper, *Rationing Health Care* (London: Croom Helm, 1975); A.J. Culyer, *Need and the National Health Service. Economics and Social Choice* (London: Martin Robertson, 1976); V.R. Fuchs, *Who Shall Live? Health, Economics and Social Choice* (New York: Basic Books, 1974); and F. Hirsch, *Social Limits to Growth* (London: Routledge and Kegan Paul, 1977).

20. A.L. Cochrane, *Effectiveness and Efficiency: Random Reflections on Health Services* (London: Nuffield Provincial Hospitals Tru•., 1972); C. Dollery, *The End of an Age of Optimism* (London: Nuffield Provincial Hospitals Trust, 1978); and T. McKeown, *The Role of Medicine: Dream, Mirage or Nemesis* (London: Nuffield Provincial Hospitals Trust, 1976). See also, for strategic analysis in individual countries: J.G. Freyman, *The American Health Care System: Its Genesis and Trajectory* (Baltimore, Md.: Williams and Wilkins, 1974); B.S. Hetzel, *Health and Australian Society* (Harmandsworth, England, and Ringwood, Victoria, Australia: Penguin, 1974); J.H. Knowles, ed., *Doing Better and Feeling Worse: Health in the United States* (New York: W.W. Norton, 1977); M. Lalonde, *A New Perspective on the Health of Canadians* (Ottawa: Government of Canada, 1974); and S. Sax, *Medical Care in the Melting Pot: An Australian Review* (Sydney: Angus and Robertson, 1972).

21. F. Roberts, *The Cost of Health* (London: Turnstile Press, 1952).

22. F. Roberts, *Cost of Health*, p. 152.

23. J.R. Seale, "A General Theory of National Expenditure on Medical Care," *Lancet*, 10 October 1959; and "Fixed Costs in The Health Service," *Lancet*, 24 September 1960.

24. See, for example: D.A. Ehrlich, ed., *The Health Care Cost Explosion: Which Way Now?* (Bern: Hans Huber, 1975); and T. Hu, ed., *International Health Costs and Expenditures*, DHEW Publication no. (NIH) 76-1067, Washington, D.C., 1976.

25. H. Hiatt, "Protecting the Medical Commons: Who Is Responsible?" *New England Journal of Medicine* (July 1975).

26. J. Tudor Hart, "The Inverse Care Law," *Lancet*, 27 February 1971.

27. J.P. Newhouse, "Medical-Care Expenditure: A Cross-National Survey," *The Journal of Human Resources* 12, no. 1 (Winter 1977): 115-125.

28. A. L. Cochrane, A.S. St. Leger and F. Moore, "Health Service 'Input' and Mortality 'Output' in Developed Countries," *Journal of Epidemiology and Community Health* 32 (1978):200-205.

29. R. Maxwell, *Health Care: The Growing Dilemma*, 2d ed. (New York: McKinsey and Company, 1975).

30. J. Le Grand, "The Distribution of Public Expenditure: The Case of Health Care," *Economica* 45 (May 1978):125-142.

31. J.P. Bunker, "Surgical Manpower: A Comparison of Operations and Surgeons in the United States and in England and Wales," *New England Journal of Medicine* 282 (1977):135; J.P. Bunker, B.A. Barnes, and F. Mosteller, eds. *Costs, Risks and Benefits of Surgery* (New York: Oxford University Press, 1977).

32. For the inequality of geographic distribution in France see: P. Cornillot and P. Bonamour, chapter titled "France" in *Health Services Prospects*, edited by I. Douglas-Wilson and G. McLachlan (London: Lancet and Nuffield, 1973); L.Lebart, S. Sandier, and T. Tonnellier, "Aspects Géographiques du Système des Soins Médicaux," *Consommation— Annales du Credoc* (Paris, 1974); H. Faure, S. Sandier and F. Tonnelier, *Analyse Régionale des Relations entre l'Offre et la Consommation de Soins Médicaux (secteur privé)* (Paris: Credoc, 1977). For geographic inequality as a more general phenomenon, not only in health services, see D.M. Smith, *Where the Grass is Greener: Living in an Unequal World* (Harmandsworth: Penguin, 1979).

33. See, for example, T. McKeown, *Role of Medicine* [20].

34. See A.L. Cochrane, *Effectiveness and Efficiency* [20].

35. The literature on health indicators is already large enough to warrant a separate bibliography and will become much larger. There are substantial differences in the conceptual approaches of different groups of researchers. I am grateful for guidance by Dr. R.M. Rosser in a recent, as yet unpublished, review of the literature, which was presented to the European workshop on health indicators at a meeting at York in January 1980. Among the main pieces to date, representing the principal schools of thought, are: W.I. Card, M. Rusenkiewicz, and C.I. Phillips, "Utility Estimates of a Set of States of Health" *Methods of Information in Medicine* 16 (1977):168; M.K. Chen and B.E. Bryant, "The Measurement of Health—A Critical and Selective Overview," *International Journal of Epidemiology* 4 (1975):257-264; M.K. Chen, "The K Index: A Proxy Measure of Health Care Quality," *Health Services Research* 11 (1976):452-462; M.M. Chen, J.W. Bush, and D.L. Patrick, "Social Indicators for Health Planning and Policy Analysis," *Policy Science* 6 (1975):71-89; C.L. Chiang and R.D. Cohen, "How to Measure Health: A Stochastic Model for an Index of Health," *International Journal of Epidemiology* 2 (1973):7-13; A.J. Culyer, R.J. Lavers, and A. Williams, "Social Indicators: Health," in *Social Trends, 1971*, pp. 31-42 (London: HMSO, 1971); A.J. Culyer, "Measuring Health," in *Need and the National Health Service*, A.J. Culyer, Chapter 4 (London: Martin Robertson, 1976); S. Fanshel and J.W. Bush, "A Health Status Index and its Application to Health Service Outcomes," *Operations Research* 18 (1970):1021-1066; S. Katz, A.B. Ford, R.W. Moskowitz, B.A. Jacobson, and M.W. Jaffe, "The Index

of ADL: A Standardized Measure of Biological and Psychosocial Function," *Journal of the American Medical Association* 185 (1963): 914-919; R.M. Rosser and V.C. Watts, "The Measurement of Hospital Output," *International Journal of Epidemiology* 1 (1972):361-367; R.M. Rosser and V.C. Watts, "The Measurement of Illness," *Journal of Operational Research* 29 (1978):529; R.M. Rosser and P. Kind, "A Scale of Valuations of States of Illness: A Social Consensus," *International Journal of Epidemiology* 7 (1978):347-357; G.W. Torrance, "Health Status Preferences: A Comparative Study of Three Measurement Techniques," *Socio-Economic Planning Sciences* 10 (1976): 129-136; R.G.A. Williams, M. Johnston, L.A. Willis, and A.E. Bennett, "Disability: a Model and Measurement Technique," *British Journal of Preventive and Social Medicine* 30 (1976):71-78.

36. I. Illich, *Medical Nemesis: The Expropriation of Health* (London: Calder and Boyers, 1975). He overstates the case, but raises questions that should be asked.

37. These estimates are given by J. Califano, then secretary of DHEW, in a memorandum to the president on national health insurance, dated 22 May 1978.

38. For a discussion of the issues raised by proposals to move from a taxation-funded service to financial arrangements based on insurance and charges, see A. Maynard, "Pricing, Insurance and the National Health Service," *Journal of Social Policy* 8, no. 2 (1979):157-176.

39. J.E. Powell, *Medicine and Politics: 1975 and After* (London: Pitman Medical, 1976). See particularly chapter 3 in this connection; but the whole book has remarkable insight, whatever one's view of Enoch Powell's politics.

40. S.A. Lindgren, chapter titled "Sweden" (esp. figure 8), in *Health Service Prospects*, edited by I. Douglas-Wilson and G. McLachlan (London: Lancet and Nuffield, 1973).

41. Department of Health and Social Security *A Happier Old Age* (London: HMSO, 1978. See chart D.)

42. A. Hunt, *The Elderly at Home* (London: Office of Population Censuses and Surveys, HMSO, 1978).

43. R.M. Ball, "United States Policy toward the Elderly" in *Care of the Elderly*, edited by A.N. Exton-Smith and J.G. Evans (London: Academic Press, 1977).

44. Based on A. Svanborg, chapter titled "Sweden," in *Geriatric Care in Advanced Societies*, edited by J.C. Brocklehurst (Lancaster: Medical and Technical Publishing Co., 1975). Dr. Svanborg's statistics in this chapter are primarily for those aged 70 and over. My figure is based on a reading of the chapter. If it is wrong, the error is mine; it could even be an understatement.

45. S.P. Strickland, *Politics, Science and Dread Disease: A Short History of the U.S.A. Medical Research Policy* (Cambridge, Mass.: Harvard University Press, Commonwealth Funds Publication Service, 1972).

46. W. Laing, *End Stage Renal Failure*, OHE Briefing no. 11 (London: Office of Health Economics, April 1980). Laing makes extensive and imaginative use of data from the European Dialysis and Transplant Association.

47. This is, of course, part of the Illich thesis (*Medical Nemesis* [36]). For a horrifying parable of what can be inflicted in the name of treatment, see also J.E. McClelland, in *The Health Service Administrator: Innovator or Catalyst?*, edited by L. Paine (London: King Edward's Hospital Fund, 1978), pp. 50-52.

48. B. Abel-Smith, *Value for Money in Health Services* (London: Heinemann, 1976); and "Value for Money," in *Health Care Planning*, edited by J.C.J. Burkens et al. (Amsterdam and Oxford: Excerpta Medica, 1976), pp. 37-44.

49. See *Public Expenditure on Health* [8], p.65.

50. This proposition is expounded by many health economists, perhaps most forcefully by Michael H. Cooper in *Rationing Health Care* (London: Croom Helm, 1975). In truth, the influence of physicians varies by condition, and this is well discussed by David Mechanic in *Future Issues in Health Care* (New York: Free Press, 1979), p. 38 ff. In addition, as stated by Rudolf Klein in *Complaints against Doctors* (London: Charles Knight, 1973), the medical profession has substantial political influence, not so much in dictating public policy as in defining what is politically possible.

51. M.I. Roemer, "Bed Supply and Hospital Utilization: A Natural Experiment," *Hospitals*, 1 November 1961, pp. 35-42.

52. See C.M. Saunders, ed., *The Management of Terminal Disease* (London: Edward Arnold, 1978). It is important that the hospice movement should have a much broader influence than the establishment of separate institutions called hospices. The approach is equally relevant in acute and long-stay hospitals and at home.

53. See D. Mechanic, *Future Issues in Health Care* (New York: Free Press, 1979).

Index

Abel-Smith, Brian, studies by, 4-6, 5, 8, 10-12, 14, 19-20, 35-37, 78, 111
Accidents: automobile, 106-107; prevention of, 52
Accounting procedures: national health, 2, 5; standard format for, 1, 5
Acute-care hospital beds, 11, 90
Administration: central, 93; complexities, 65; costs, 63, 93; financing, 13; flexibility, 69; health-care, 19, 26, 86; institutions and agencies, 99; of services, 100-101; and staffing requirements, 20
Administrators: governmental, 66; health-care, 10
Age and the elderly, 13, 21, 33, 39, 44, 88-90, 99, 106, 112; mortality rates, 106; residential homes for, 82, 89; services for, 92; treatment of, 100
Agencies: administration of, 99; health-insurance, 50-51; health-service-ownership, 66; and private institutions, 13; public, 97
Alcoholism and alcohol consumption, 11, 23, 52, 106; and driving, 108
Ambulatory care, 82, 97; hospital-based, 112; inpatient, 19; medical services, 7
Armed forces, medical services for, 19, 99
Australia: buildings, 80; capital expenses, 19, 21; community programs, 109; elderly in, 91; government administration, 66-69; gross national product, 21, 41, 44-45, 101; health-care expenditures, 30, 33-35, 37-39, 99; hospital expenses, 82-83, 86-99, 90; insurance programs, 62-63, 105; mortality rate, 52-56; pharmaceuticals, 78-79; physicians in, 73-74; private and public financing, 59-61; resources in, 71, 75; self-medication, 92; studies of, 12, 14; tax policies, 64-65
Automobile: accidents, 106-107; and alcohol drinking, 108
Auxiliary: nurses, 74; staffing, 20

Belgium, 77
Benefits: cash, 4, 99; pharmaceutical, 3
Birth rate, effects of, 39, 46
Borrowing and borrowers, 5
Budgets and budgetary control, 80, 103
Buildings and equipment, 20, 79-81; depreciation on, 4

Canada: administration, 66-69; annual statistics, 1; budgetary controls, 103; buildings, 80; community programs, 109; diseases in, 107; elderly in, 91;

government controls, 47, 49; gross national product, 6, 41, 44-45, 101; health-care expenditures, 30, 33-35, 37-39; hospital expenses, 82-83, 86-88, 90; insurance programs, 63; manpower, 70; medical schools, 76; mortality rate, 52-56; pharmaceuticals, 77-79; physicians, 73-74; private and public financing, 59-61; provincial taxes, 64-65; resources of, 71, 75; self-medication in, 92; studies of, 12, 14, 18
Cancer, lung, 106-107
Capital: construction, 21, 24; costs, 4, 80; expenditure, 6, 19; formation, 6, 69; interest on, 4
Cash, 100; benefits, 20, 22, 99; payments, 4, 65
Census information, use of, 97
Centralization, factor of, 64, 66, 69, 93
Centre de recherche pour l'etude et l'observation des conditions de vie (CREDOC), 2-3, 13-14, 17, 112
Ceylon, 4
Charities and charitable foundations: non-government, 67; services of, 19-20, 24, 69; and voluntary donations, 4
Chile, 4
Chronic illnesses, 39, 46, 51
Cigarette smoking, effects of, 11, 52, 108
Circulatory diseases, 107
Cochrane, Archie L., 11, 14
Communist bloc countries, 12, 35
Community: care, 57, 86, 92; health services, 48, 69, 97, 112; responsibility, 50, 66; support networks, 107, 109
Construction: capital, 21, 24; and major renovation, 80
Consumer: goods, 110; payments, 19, 64-65, 105; price indexes, 7
Control: budgetary, 103; financial, 105-107, 111; of institutions, 97; manpower, 81; price, 102; public, 107; of supplies, 13
Cost(s): administration, 63, 93; ambulance, 21, 24; capital, 4, 80; health-services, 1, 3, 81, 112; operating, 4-5; personnel, 103; traveling, 99
Cross-national: comparisons, 3-5; surveys, 7-8, 12
Czechoslovakia, 4

Data: availability, 1, 17-18, 21; collection, 12, 15, 17, 21, 100, 111-113; international, 111-113; national, 2; reliability of, 97-98
Death, 51; premature, 108; rate of, 57

175

About the Author

Robert J. Maxwell is Secretary of King Edward's Hospital Fund for London. Previously, he was Administrator to the Special Trustees for St. Thomas' Hospital, London. He received master's degrees from Oxford University and the University of Pennsylvania, and a doctorate from The London School of Economics. He is also a qualified management accountant. He became interested in international comparisons in the health-care field as a result of consulting on a series of projects for hospitals, health authorities, and governments, mainly in the developed world. He has written frequently on this topic, including *Health Care: The Growing Dilemma* (1974).